A Busy Person's Guide to a
Healthier Life

MATT DRAGON

D1496214

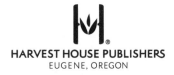

HARVEST HOUSE PUBLISHERS
EUGENE, OREGON

Cover design by Aesthetic Soup

Cover photo © 7505811966, roundex, ZinetroN, artem evdokimov / Shutterstock

This book contains stories in which people's names and some details of their situations have been changed.

A Busy Person's Guide to a Healthier Life

Copyright © 2019 Matt Dragon
Published by Harvest House Publishers
Eugene, Oregon 97408
www.harvesthousepublishers.com

ISBN 978-0-7369-7546-9 (pbk.)
ISBN 197-0-7369-7547-6 (eBook)

Library of Congress Cataloging-in-Publication Data

Names: Dragon, Matt, author.
Title: A busy person's guide to a healthier life / Matt Dragon.
Description: Eugene, Oregon : Harvest House Publishers, [2019] | Includes
  bibliographic references.
Identifiers: LCCN 2018038717 (print) | LCCN 2018047373 (ebook) | ISBN
  9780736975476 (ebook) | ISBN 9780736975469 (pbk.) | ISBN 1970736975476
  (eBook)
Subjects: LCSH: Health—Popular works. | Health behavior—Popular works. |
  Health—Religious aspects—Christianity.
Classification: LCC RA776 (ebook) | LCC RA776 .D785 2019 (print) | DDC
  613.2—dc23
LC record available at https://lccn.loc.gov/2018038717

Printed in the United States of America

19 20 21 22 23 24 25 26 27 / BP-GL / 10 9 8 7 6 5 4 3 2 1

Contents

Part 2: Exercise and Fitness

Part 3: Rest, Recover, Recharge

A Note to the Reader

This book provides advice and information on exercise, nutrition, rest, and general fitness. It has been written for your personal knowledge and to help you become a healthier person. It is not intended to replace advice from your physician or other health professionals. This book's contents should be used to supplement, not replace, regular care and personalized advice from qualified medical professionals.

Consult with your physician or other health practitioner if you have specific questions and concerns. Thorough efforts have been made to ensure the accuracy of the information in this book as of the publication date.

Foreword

Matt Dragon's mindset and approach to health, fitness, nutrition, training, and recovery allow him to provide much-needed nuggets of truth in an age of fluff, glitter, and celebrity fitness gurus.

Matt is a military veteran and world-class athlete even though he's in his early forties now. That's why I value and respect his advice. As a competitive athlete myself, I have found that Matt's advice helps me physically, mentally, and spiritually. This guy knows his stuff!

Whether you are a professional-caliber athlete or just a man or woman hoping to improve your health so you can enjoy a long and happy life, this book will give you time-tested, easy-to-understand advice that will add great value to your life no matter how old or how young you are.

Read this book. Apply it. You will be a healthier person as a result, and that good health will enhance all facets of your life!

Gabriel Johnson is a five-time American Grappling Federation jiujitsu champion, a two-time absolute champion of the American Grappling Federation, and a silver medalist at the US National Championships of the International Brazilian Jiu-Jitsu Federation.

Introduction

Good morning! It might not be morning for you, but it is for me. I have just finished my morning routine. I drank a large glass of water and then did some light calisthenics. I enjoyed a favorite beverage—water with a little honey, cinnamon, and lemon. I ate a light breakfast followed by a protein shake.

Now I am going to write for a while before taking a long walk. I am giving you a glimpse into how I live every day as a very busy person trying his best to stay healthy and fit. As you will see in the pages of this book, I live what I write.

I am not writing about how to have perfect health. This book is not about how you can have six-pack abs or bulging biceps. When I wrote my first eBook, I posted a picture of myself shirtless. I was not in the best shape of my life, but I wasn't in the worst shape of my life either. I am not a model, and I am certainly not a trained photographer. I didn't wear any makeup. I didn't use trick lighting or filters. I wanted to show myself as I really was. There will be no such pictures of me in this book, but I do want to share an accurate description of my lifestyle.

Here's a bit more about who I really am. I started competing in sports at age 9. I started *training* for sports at 11. In high school, I competed in basketball, football, and track. At 17, I traveled to the Philippines to play basketball on a short-term mission trip. At 21, I was hiking and climbing in Nepal.

Later, I joined the United States Air Force, and I worked in signals intelligence for several years. Since then, I have worked as a government contractor, serving in Iraq and Afghanistan. I wish I could tell you more about my government work, but I can't. I'm sure you understand why.

I am also a Level 1 US Olympic weight-lifting coach, and I hold certifications from John Davies, the creator of Renegade Training, and Mike Mahler, the internationally known strength coach and kettlebell instructor.

I like superheroes, dogs (more accurately, animals in general), my friends and family, wine and beer (in moderation), roller coasters, physical and mental challenges, leather seats, and books (lots and lots of books), just to name a few things.

Here's why I am writing this book. According to the Centers for Disease Control and Prevention, more than 70 percent of US adults over age 20 are overweight or obese.[1] Now, I have never been obese, but I have become too fat for my own comfort level. A few years ago, I looked in the mirror and saw that I had developed love handles. That was enough for me. I felt disappointed in myself.

How had things gone wrong for me? I wanted to compete in strongman competitions, like the ones you might have seen on TV. I felt that I needed to gain weight to compete effectively. I wanted to be one of those 300-pound monsters who can tow an airplane. I am six feet three inches tall, and I usually weigh about 220 pounds.

I bulked up to 250 pounds, and people started asking me if I was on steroids. (I wasn't.) I didn't feel like a behemoth, but I realized that too much of my new poundage was fat. My joints started to ache because of the added bulk. Looking back, I realize that I could have been much smarter about adding weight. It's one of the health lessons I learned the hard way.

I am confessing this mistake because this book is about real life, not an unreachable ideal. As a high school football player, I was recruited by some Division 1 schools until a knee injury ended my career. (More about that in chapter 36, "Conquer Injuries.") If you are a former athlete, I hope my experience will encourage you to get back in the game at some level. But this is not a book for athletes only.

---

[1] Centers for Disease Control and Prevention, National Center for Health Statistics, "Obesity and Overweight," www.cdc.gov/nchs/fastats/obesity-overweight.htm.

I enjoy serving and helping all kinds of people. That's why I served my country in the air force. That's why I became a certified Olympic weight-lifting instructor and a personal trainer.

I also love challenging myself. I am currently competing in Brazilian jiujitsu (BJJ), and I am loving the process of learning a new sport. When I started, I was being submitted by 125-pound females, but that was okay by me. I felt privileged to be competing with empowered women. What's more, there is a saying in BJJ: "Either you win or you learn." Those words contain so much wisdom. Change your definition of success and you will change the way you see life. Sometimes when you lose, you win.

I have also taken up longboarding in recent months. So when I challenge you to try new things to improve your health, please know that I live by that advice. I wouldn't encourage you to try anything I wasn't willing to try myself.

Most of what I share in this book is based on my personal experiences. I want to share what I have learned as a member of the air force and as an athlete, coach, and trainer. I particularly want to note my mistakes and what I have learned from them.

Today I am not a perfect physical specimen, but I am healthier than I once was. Like most people, I want to be fit and healthy. When I fall short of that goal, I become unhappy. This morning, I am relatively pleased with my overall fitness and general health. I am aware of areas in which I could improve, but I am happy with who Matt Dragon is—physically, mentally, and spiritually. I pray I can help you feel the same about yourself.

Part I

Diet and Nutrition

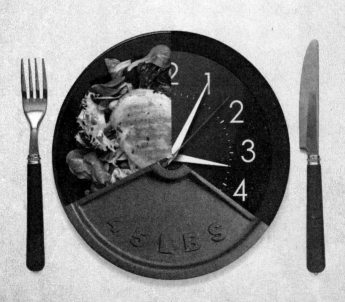

1

Begin Well

As I mentioned in the introduction, I am a coach and fitness trainer who currently "rolls" in Brazilian jiujitsu. However, I don't know my own body-fat percentage. I will write about some of the measurement methods in chapter 26, "Don't Fight a Losing Battle," but I caution the people I train to avoid becoming obsessed about their percentages.

Many of the methods can be unreliable anyway—for example, it's easy to cheat when measuring skin folds with calipers—but that doesn't mean we shouldn't track our progress. I recommend taking pictures of yourself (or having someone snap pics for you) every two to three weeks. Try to get your pics in the morning before you eat or drink anything.

As for measuring yourself, I suggest getting simple tape measurements of your upper torso, stomach (both upper abs and belly button area), hips, calves, neck, and upper arms.

If this sounds too cumbersome or unpleasant, here is one of the most accurate fitness trackers of all: How does your favorite pair of jeans fit? Believe it or not, this is one of the best ways to measure your progress. We can see (or *think* we see) signs of progress in our faces and limbs, but often, the gut and the butt are the last to go.

During a tour of duty in Afghanistan, I was minding my own business when a colleague decided to sit down nearby and educate me about nutrition. Roger was about six feet tall, and I estimated he weighed about 350 pounds. Let's just say most of that weight was not muscle. I listened patiently to Roger for several minutes.

I think he began to sense my skepticism about his advice because he interrupted the lesson to say, "I know, right? Look at me. Who am I to be giving *you* advice? But I want you to understand that I really do know what I am talking about. I know what I *should* be doing with diet and exercise and all that—I just don't have the time for it."

Next, Roger elaborated on why he was too busy to get fit and healthy. As he talked, he finished his first can of Coke and started on his second. Only ten minutes had elapsed since he approached me.

Roger occasionally digressed from the health advice to tell me about the many TV shows he watched regularly. I wondered how he found time for all that TV but none for exercising.

I share this story because too many of us take advice from people who don't practice what they preach. Would you take financial advice from a pauper? Would you read a marriage book from an author who has endured three bitter divorces and is now single?

There is a reason this book is titled *A Busy Person's Guide to a Healthier Life*. I hear excuses all the time, sometimes from my own lips. Do any of these statements sound familiar?

- I just don't have the time to exercise.
- Healthful foods are too expensive.
- I can't get motivated to eat right or exercise.
- Too much of today's health advice is contradictory. I don't know whom to believe.
- I have a spouse, kids, a job, a dog, and a cat. I don't have time for *anything* else in my life.
- I travel all the time. There's no way to maintain any kind of routine or program.
- I injured myself several years ago, and I can't really do any sports or fitness activities anymore.

I understand these challenges. Like you, my life is hectic. I am looking at my United Airlines mileage total right now—it's up to 138,441.

I have four kids. During the past seven years, I have usually worked twelve hours a day, seven days a week.

Much of my work has been in Iraq and Afghanistan. As you might have seen on TV, the life of a government contractor in the war-ravaged Middle East is not one of personal trainers, state-of-the art fitness equipment, and personal chefs.

I have known the heartbreak of divorce. Perhaps you have too.

I have been seriously injured, and I deal with those complications every day. Again, you may relate.

We are all busy, imperfect people facing many challenges. But I am here to tell you that exercising, eating right, and learning how to rest and recharge my body and soul have helped me get through many of life's hardships. Being healthy helps keep us sane when life becomes overwhelming. Our bodies and minds need a release. Our spirits need a release. And I believe an over-reliance on TV and electronic gadgets is *not* a release. So much of today's entertainment is toxic. In chapter 45, I encourage you to take an occasional "technology fast." I hope you will embrace that challenge. You'll be amazed at how much better you'll feel.

While we are on the subject of technology…have you noticed that the same people who claim they have no time to exercise or to eat right can tell you all about their favorite TV shows, apps, video games, or fantasy sports leagues?

You *can* find the time to make a fresh start and make the principles in this book work for you. For example, TV doesn't have to be an excuse or a roadblock. Neither does business travel. Last night, I worked out in my hotel room while half-watching a reality survival show on TV. I can't recommend the show I watched, but it did help me pass the time while I did some light calisthenics and equipment-free exercises, like push-ups, sit-ups, planks, lunges, and burpees.

The key to creating a healthier life for yourself and those you love is to start looking for *opportunities*, not excuses. For example, if you are staying in a high-rise hotel for a business trip or vacation, take the stairs as much as you can and avoid standing around waiting for the elevator.

> The key to creating a healthier life for yourself and those you love is to start looking for *opportunities*, not excuses.

Does your hotel have long hallways? Pace off the distance and then walk a mile. (It's roughly 1,760 steps if you're a long strider.) You can walk while making phone calls, checking your voice mail, or rehearsing for your upcoming business presentation.

Look for opportunities to do something positive for your health *every day*. It might be skipping dessert at the business dinner. It might be trying your morning cup of coffee *without* the two packets of sugar or the corn-syrup-laden nondairy creamer.

You may be dealing with the long-term effects of illness or injury. You might have had a passion (like football and strongman competitions were for me), but you can no longer do those activities.

That's okay. Find something else. Some martial arts studios have one- or two-week trials. I found that I could lose fat and build strength and flexibility with Brazilian jiujitsu. I'm only a blue belt right now, but I hope to earn a black belt someday. And I am enjoying the challenge of taking up a new sport in my forties.

Additionally, I find some way to strength train at least three times a week even if I don't have access to free weights or weight machines. As we'll explore later, you don't necessarily need weights to build strength and muscle.

In fact, if you are passionate about a sport or a form of exercise, but you are still unhappy with your weight or fitness level, strength training is probably the missing link.

Or you might need to add some cardio work. One simple solution is to find a way to add an hour of walking to your daily schedule. Walk to work if you can. If you're going shopping, park at the far end of the parking lot. Recently when I was in a big-box store, I took ten minutes to walk around the perimeter of the store. I took a second lap, giving me twenty minutes toward my one-hour goal for the day.

On the diet and nutrition front, most of us can rack up big improvements by paying closer attention to what we put into our bodies. How many sodas do you drink per week? Sodas add nothing good to our diets. (You might gather that I am not a fan of soft drinks. You'll learn more about that later.)

How much alcohol do you drink in an average week? How often do you raid the snack drawer at home or the treat jar at work?

As we close this chapter, take a minute to compile a simple list of five things you can do to start getting healthier *right now*. Commit to doing these things in the coming week. Here is one of my lists.

1. Walk an hour a day.
2. Eat lean protein at every meal.
3. Stop drinking soda and replace it with water.
4. Avoid white bread.
5. Weight train.

Once you have finished your list, pick the first thing to do. Then do it. Start right now. In fact, if you can, stop reading this book and tackle that first task. As a trainer, I know that when people sign up for a training program with me, they often start exercising *before* their first appointment. Why? Because they took that first action—making the appointment—and things snowballed from there.

Start taking action and watch your life change.

I read a lot—philosophy books, business books, self-help books from successful people who walk the walk. They all share a common theme: Do something *now*. It doesn't have to be perfect for you to begin well.

Imagine you have a bow and arrow and are shooting at a target. Look where you want the arrow to go and let loose. You can adjust your aim on subsequent shots.

I know that this advice might sound counterintuitive. Most of us have been taught "Plan your work and then work your plan." In most cases, that's helpful advice. But my personal experience and the experiences of many, many others have led me to change my tune when it comes to health and fitness. I have seen too many people get stuck at the blueprint phase.

So back to my arrow analogy. You will accomplish nothing if you spend too much time calculating the wind speed and target distance or worrying about how you look with a bow in your hands. Inaction gets you nowhere. Clinging to bad habits moves you further from your goals.

But as long as you are trying, there is hope. I promise you that.

2

You Are What You Eat!

Does this chapter title sound like good news or bad news? Your answer probably says a lot about your current eating habits. We've all been there—feeling hungry enough to eat just about anything, and the handiest option is an unhealthy combination of artery-clogging trans fats, empty calories, and high-fructose corn syrup. Then, after polishing off the jumbo order of fries or a half-dozen grocery store cookies, remorse sets in, right along with indigestion. After all, who feels happy when his stomach looks and feels like an overinflated beach ball?

Like a car, we run smoother and faster when we get the right fuel. We don't need a degree in nutrition to realize that appropriate portions and good food choices make us feel energized and satisfied. Lousy choices do the opposite. By filling ourselves with empty calories that eventually leave us hungry (and leave our bodies craving some *real* nutrition), we encourage overeating. This, in turn, causes us to avoid the scale, the mirror, and our favorite snug-fitting blue jeans.

> We are complex beings with physical bodies that house mental, emotional, and spiritual functions. So we treat our hearts, minds, and spirits well (or badly) by the way we fill our bodies.

But much more than self-esteem is at stake here. As humans, we are complex beings with physical bodies that house mental, emotional, and spiritual functions. So we treat our hearts, minds, and spirits well (or badly) by the way we fill our bodies. We consume to satisfy our taste buds and growling stomachs, but we influence much more in the process. Eating plenty of raw fruits and vegetables, tree nuts, whole grains, and good fats (such as olive oil, fish oil, or flax oil) provides a deep sense of health and well-being, which is ultimately more satisfying than the initial rush provided by a bite of some sugary, preservative-filled cupcake.

And eating the good stuff *before* anything else leaves little room to be tempted by worthless calories. (We'll dive deeper into this concept in an upcoming chapter.)

We are happier creatures with sharper minds, healthier bodies, and satisfied spirits when we feast on excellent food. Next time you refuel, reach for a fresh piece of fruit or a handful of raw nuts. You're bound to feel content in body and soul. You'll have no guilt to weigh you down. Instead, happiness is yours knowing you've given your body what it truly needs.

3

Eat Your Way from Fat to Fit

In part 1, we're focusing on diet and nutrition because what you put into your body will set the tone for your life. Even if you have great exercise habits and get plenty of sleep every night, you can't ignore your diet and expect to reach your fitness goals. It's a key to your success. You simply can't outrun, out-lift, out-train, or even out-pray a bad diet.

Imagine this book's three parts ("Diet and Nutrition"; "Exercise and Fitness"; and "Rest, Recover, and Recharge") as the three legs of a stool. If one leg is wobbly, broken, or missing entirely, you can guess what will happen.

Here are a few key dietary truths I have learned through many years as an athlete, military veteran, coach, and trainer.

First, beware of carbs. This is one of those cases in which you *can* believe much of what you are reading and hearing in the media. Carbohydrates, especially simple carbs (as opposed to complex carbs), make you fat. The carbs you ingest but don't use for energy are stored as fat. I'll explain how this happens: When we are eating wisely and exercising, the carbs we eat are turned into *glycogen*, a stored form of glucose that serves as fuel for our muscles. But if we ingest too many carbs or don't use our muscles, that potential fuel ends up being stored as fat.

Too many carbs also result in inflammation. You might have seen a trend toward anti-inflammatory diets, and there is a good reason for this. Inflammation is linked to almost every disease known to humanity.

Second, eat lean, fresh meat as often as possible (or lean, nonmeat protein if you are a vegetarian or vegan). By fresh, I mean unprocessed and free of various additives and flavor enhancers. And it's okay to eat meat with fat in it. Eating fat doesn't necessarily make you fat. Trans fats are what make you gain weight, and most trans fats are associated with carbs, not leaner cuts of fresh meat.

Here is a fact many people don't realize: Your body needs a certain amount of fat to function properly. If you don't provide those fats through your diet, your body will store fat. I know this sounds counterintuitive, but it's true. Avoiding healthy fat can make you fatter.

> It sounds counterintuitive, but avoiding healthy fat in your diet can make you fatter.

Here's another important dietary principle to remember: Carbs tend to make us hungrier, but fat tends to satiate us. In other words, if your body doesn't get the fat and protein it needs, it signals your brain to eat more. And if you continue to eat carbs, you are not giving your body what it needs. So more signals bombard your brain—"Eat, eat, eat!"—and the unhealthy cycle repeats itself.

Remember when we used to eat eggs and a reasonable amount of bacon for breakfast? That's a breakfast loaded with protein and some of the fat our bodies need. As you'll read more than once in this book, I am a big fan of eggs. They are good for your brain because they provide folate, choline, and B vitamins—all important ingredients for brain and body health and function.

Eggs also provide vitamins A and D and iodine, a necessary nutrient. Compare the nutrient-per-gram content of eggs and lean meat to almost any vegetable you can think of. You might be surprised by the results.

Here's just one example, courtesy of one of my favorite websites, TwoFoods, which compares the nutritional value of many different kinds of food.

According to this site, a 100-gram serving of carrots provides 41 calories, 9.6 grams of carbs, .24 grams of fat, and .93 grams of protein.

Meanwhile, a 100-gram serving of hard-boiled egg contains 155 calories but only 1.1 grams of carbs. The fat content is higher, 10.6 grams, but this is not trans fat. And when it comes to protein, it's no contest. The egg packs 12.58 grams of protein, more than 12 times the carrots' protein content.

You have probably heard terms like "essential fatty acids," "essential amino acids," and "essential proteins." But have you ever heard a doctor or nutritionist discuss "essential carbohydrates"? That is because they don't exist.

Yes, I know carbs tend to taste good, but your body *needs* protein and fat. Feed your body what it needs. Your taste buds will follow. Remember, we are fearfully and wonderfully made! Our diets should honor this truth.

4

Set Smart Priorities

A time-management expert faced a group of business students. He set a one-gallon glass jar on a table and then emptied a bag containing a dozen fist-sized rocks. He placed each rock in the jar and then asked his audience, "Is this jar full?"

The business students agreed it was. The expert raised his eyebrows and reached under the table for a bucket of gravel. He dumped it in and then shook the jar until the gravel settled among the rocks. He asked the group again, "Now is the jar full?"

By this time, most of the class was onto him. "I don't think it's truly full," one student called out.

The expert grabbed a bag of sand and poured it into the jar. A few shakes later, the sand had sifted its way among the rocks and gravel. "What about now?" he asked. "Is it full?"

"No!" the class answered.

The presenter took the bucket that once held the gravel. He filled it with water from a nearby drinking fountain. He added the water to the jar until the liquid reached the brim. "What do you learn from this?" he asked his audience.

One student raised her hand. "No matter how full your schedule is, you can always fit a few more things into it," she offered.

"No, no, no," the speaker replied, shaking his head. "You're missing it. Imagine how things would have gone if I put the water, sand, and gravel in *before* the big rocks. How do you think that would have worked out? Think about it—if you don't put the big rocks in first, you'll never be able to squeeze them in later."

Think about this episode in relation to your diet and your general health right now. Every single day, you face the challenge of setting smart priorities. When it comes to diet and nutrition, what are the big rocks in your life? Eating more fresh vegetables and fruit? Cutting back on processed sugars? Starting each day with a healthful breakfast? Make sure you put those in your jar first, or the smaller stuff will crowd them out.

This principle applies to exercise and to rest and recovery as well. As you strive to become a healthier person, I encourage you to picture that big glass jar. Are you filling it wisely with your priorities in mind? If so, great job! If not, it's not too late to dump out the sand, gravel, and water and start over.

> Our greatest danger in life is in permitting the
> urgent things to crowd out the important.
> CHARLES E. HUMMEL

5

Make Your Home a Food-Smart Zone

If you travel a lot, as I do, you've seen that not all hotels are created equal. That's why I love finding a hotel room that has been thoughtfully designed with an ergonomically functional desk chair, adjustable lighting, a smart TV with streaming services and internet access, and plenty of charging stations and electrical outlets.

I appreciate hotels that are *traveler smart*. They make my time away from home more effective and enjoyable.

In a similar vein, I encourage you to make your home (especially your kitchen) *food smart*. This will take some effort, but you are worth it. No matter how you might be feeling about yourself as you read this book, you are a unique and valuable person created by God. There is a unique purpose and plan for your life.

With this important fact in mind, let's look at ways to ensure your home or apartment is designed for dietary success.

First, think "homemade" when you stock and arrange your kitchen and pantry. (Chapter 6, "Be a Smart Grocery Shopper," will help.)

You probably know that eating out or ordering in often means consuming too much fat, salt, and sugar. By preparing more meals at home, you can control what's in your food and save money at the same time.

I know that many people don't have the time or expertise to cook full-course meals from scratch every night. Fortunately, you don't have to. Instead, consider these four ideas.

1. Cook in large batches and divide them into smaller servings. This tip can be a game changer, especially if you live alone or perhaps with one other person. "Batch cooking" can be an efficient and delicious way to go. I have seen people make a few pots of soup or a few casseroles, and before long, they were off and running. I know a young millennial woman who started making a batch of breakfast burritos at the start of the week. She and her husband eat a few of the burritos right away. Others are refrigerated for later in the week, and yet more are frozen for use later.

Even if you live by yourself in a small apartment, don't be afraid to create a large batch of your favorite healthful recipes. It won't take long to learn which ones make the best leftovers. Soups and chilis are big favorites for me. Like my friends' burritos, your extra soup, chili, or stew can be refrigerated or frozen for later use.

If you need to, invest in a few storage containers and keep a supply of ziplock bags on hand. Once you have a ready supply of "batched dishes," you won't have to face that daily challenge of figuring out what to eat for breakfast, lunch, and dinner.

Keep in mind that batching works for all meals as well as snacks. I will bake oatmeal in a 9 × 13 pan and reheat the leftovers later in the week. Healthy egg casseroles are also great for multiple breakfasts. While we are on the subject of eggs, boil a bunch of them at a time and refrigerate what you don't eat right away. Hard-boiled eggs are a fine grab-and-go breakfast as well as a healthy snack option. (Whether peeled or unpeeled, hard-boiled eggs will keep for about a week in your refrigerator.)

2. *Make the freezer your friend.* I tell people all the time, "Your freezer is more than an ice cream stash." Freezing food saves time and money. (We Americans throw out too much food. It's like throwing away nutrition and money at the same time.) Label your containers so you know what you are dealing with. (Use this for the fridge food too. Put a name and a date on everything. This is one reason I favor storing my hard-boiled eggs unpeeled. I can write my info right on the shells.)

I love to make a big batch of pasta sauce in my slow cooker. I refrigerate some of it and freeze the rest. By the way, if you are wondering how long you can freeze or refrigerate food, I recommend sites like

StillTasty, which allows you to type in a food item and get recommendations. For example, you will learn that refrigerated pasta sauce with meat will last three or four days in your fridge but up to six months in the freezer. (Quick tip: In terms of food safety, most frozen foods have an almost indefinite life-span. However, freezer burn and general lack of taste and quality can become issues after several months.)

If you need ideas for "batch cooking," Pinterest has all kinds of meal suggestions and tips. BudgetBytes is another useful site. Even a basic internet search will get you started.

Remember that the freezer works great for side dishes too. I like to freeze fresh vegetables and fruit, especially before winter arrives and it's harder to find certain varieties of fresh produce. I also like to freeze a few smoothies. I can grab one for a quick breakfast or a midday energy boost.

And we can't leave this topic without addressing desserts. Have you ever made cookie dough and baked all of it (or baked most of it and eaten the rest raw)? It's hard to limit portions when it comes to cookies, especially when they are hot from the oven. That's why, when I prepare cookie dough, I immediately set aside at least half. I roll this dough into small balls and freeze them in a flat storage container. This keeps the cookies from sticking together. When I'm ready to bake those extra balls of dough, I can grab a reasonable number. This is a smart way to make sure your after-dinner cookie consumption is limited to two or three cookies, not five or six. It usually takes about a half hour for those frozen cookie balls to thaw and cook, so I find I am more thoughtful about my consumption. I protect myself from cookie binges—you can too.

3. Embrace the power of one-ingredient foods. When you are trying to eat healthfully but you also value convenience, you can't beat this food category. By one-ingredient foods, I am talking about simple items that require little to no preparation: carrot sticks, celery sticks, fresh fruit, pea pods, and the aforementioned hard-boiled eggs. A lot of people assume that healthful eating is time-consuming and complicated.

Of course, the opposite is true. There are so many great choices that are easy.

This category of food makes wonderful snacks or on-the-go meals. One-ingredient foods are also an excellent way to incorporate something healthful into your sit-down meals. For example, consider adding a fresh fruit to breakfast, lunch, or dinner. And I don't mean a fruit salad or fancy mixed fruit; I am talking about eating half a grapefruit at breakfast, an apple with your lunch, or carrot sticks with dinner.

It's so easy. Just rinse a few grapes or cut up an apple and you have a tasty and healthful side dish.

Here's something else I love about one-ingredient foods: Cooking healthful meals (especially those your family will actually eat) can be a challenge. You might have a few flops along the way. But it's hard to mess up rinsing some grapes, peeling an orange, or slicing a grapefruit in half.

Keep these one-derful foods in mind at snack time too. Instead of grabbing a candy bar from your snack drawer, opt for a banana or clementine instead.

4. Tempt-proof your kitchen. If you're like me and always on the go, you tend to eat what is most convenient. Time often seems to be the ruling factor. How many times have you eaten a snack you knew wasn't healthy just because it was handy? You are not alone. One study revealed that we are three times more likely to eat the first food we see than to reach for the fifth item that catches our eye. And how many of us won't even take the time to look beyond that first thing that captures our notice?[1]

> If you're like me and always on the go, you tend to eat what is most convenient. Time often seems to be the ruling factor. How many times have you eaten a snack you knew wasn't healthy just because it was handy?

[1] Brian Wansink, *Mindless Eating: Why We Eat More Than We Think* (New York, NY: Bantam Books, 2010); cited in Amanda Chan, "We Are More Likely to Eat What We See First," *HuffPost,* December 6, 2017, https://www.huffingtonpost.com/2011/09/29/see-first-eat-visible-food_n_984004.html.

What are your trigger foods? For some, it's potato chips. If there's a bowl or bag of them on the kitchen counter, it's game over. For others, it's chocolate chip cookies, whether the actual cookies or just the dough. (That's one reason I recommend freezing extra dough.) I recommend making your trigger foods hard to reach. Don't put them at eye level in your pantry or refrigerator.

In other words, keep a bowl of fruit (apples, oranges, bananas, and so on) on the kitchen counter instead of cookies, chips, or candy. Remember, you are most likely to grab what's easy, so make the healthy stuff the easiest to access.

6

Be a Smart Grocery Shopper

The quest for a healthier diet begins at the grocery store or farmers market. Buy your food with a plan. Make a list and stick to it. I tell people all the time, "Grocery shop like you mean it." Here are a few suggestions for you.

Make Your Cart Colorful

This doesn't mean you should stock up on M&M's or Skittles. I'm talking about fruits and vegetables. Your cart should look like a rainbow of healthy stuff. Before you get to the checkout line, ask yourself, "Is there a wide sampling of colors here?" This is important because many fruits and veggies get their colors from the various micronutrients and antioxidants they contain. So the wider the variety of colors in your cart, the better the chances that you are covering your nutritional bases.

I put this suggestion first because I encourage you, in the spirit of chapter 4, to head for the produce section first. Make fruits and veggies your "big rocks"—the things you put in your "jar" first. Buy fresh produce for the week ahead. Get some leafy greens and thin-skinned berries for the early part of the week, and restock your pantry with potatoes and apples if needed. By the way, potatoes often get a bad rap for being too starchy. However, one russet potato has only 150 calories and is loaded with potassium. In fact, the average russet packs more than twice the potassium of a small- to medium-sized banana. Potatoes are inexpensive, and they don't have to be deep-fried to taste good. Try sautéing potatoes with spinach and topping them with a bit of fresh parmesan cheese.

I like to stock up on berries during the summer, when they are inexpensive and plentiful. Berries are great snacks. They can add nutrition and flavor to almost any meal, especially breakfast. Stir them into Greek yogurt, cold cereal, or oatmeal. Freeze what you don't use right away. I love going to my freezer and grabbing some frozen blueberries to stir into pancake batter or blend into a smoothie.

Be a Protein Pro

I have already praised the protein found in lean meats. Here are a few other great choices: Eggs are loaded with protein, and they are a go-to ingredient for many of my meals and snacks. I love breakfast scrambles featuring eggs, turkey bacon, onions, and spinach—and not just for breakfast. I also like to slice hard-boiled eggs and add them to a salad. And as we have already seen, hard-boiled eggs make perfect on-the-go snacks.

Frozen shrimp offer another great way to give meals and snacks a protein boost. I love to have some shrimp on hand to pop into a stir-fry or fold into a pasta sauce. Or you can defrost some (cooked) shrimp the night before and toss them into a salad.

Go Greek with Your Yogurt

Most of the nonfat varieties of Greek yogurt are still thick and creamy. This stuff makes a great dip, and it's a smart substitute for mayonnaise in creamy salad dressings.

Go with the Whole Grain

If grains are part of your diet, make sure they are whole grains, minimally processed. Try replacing white rice or pasta with bulgur, farro, barley, and quinoa. (Of course, quinoa isn't really a grain, but it's often prepared like one, and it's a super complex carbohydrate.) These high-fiber foods can be mixed with cooked veggies for a warm salad or tossed with herbs and some cheese to make an appealing, multi-textured side dish.

Go International

When it comes to condiments, Americans tend to make the same old choices: mustard, ketchup, mayo, and salt. Often, too much salt. I encourage you to visit the international or "world foods" aisle of your favorite store to discover some new flavors. International condiments often pack less corn syrup and fewer fillers and strange chemicals. Here are a few suggestions.

- *Hoisin sauce.* This thick and flavorful Chinese staple is a mixture of soybeans, garlic, chili peppers, and assorted spices. Hoisin sauce makes a tasty veggie stir-fry. I also use it instead of barbecue sauce when grilling chicken or ribs.

- *Curry paste.* Try this in noodle or vegetable dishes. I also like to stir it into soup stock or coconut milk when making a stew or soup.

- *Soy sauce.* I recommend the low-sodium variety of this sauce for making dips, rice side dishes, or vegetable stir-fries.

- *Sriracha.* If you have a taste for the spicy, try this crimson Asian sauce on your eggs, burgers, or salad dressing. You can also mix it with mayo for a spicy sandwich spread.

- *Harissa.* This North African spicy sauce is a combo of garlic, chilies, coriander, cumin, and a few other spices. It is wonderfully flavorful and adds a savory kick to couscous, quinoa, vegetables, and stews. I sometimes add a couple spoonfuls of harissa to a favorite soup or stew recipe, and it's almost like I have created a whole new dish.

Try some new foods and spices in your effort to eat more healthfully. Some people associate "healthful" with boring or tasteless. That certainly does not have to be the case. Adding a few exotic flavors to your meals and snacks can help you stick with your new eating habits.

7

Try a Food Switch

One key to eating more healthfully is to make it an adventure, a quest. I encourage you to have fun with the process. Be creative. Experiment. One of the best ways to do this is to challenge yourself or your family members to a *food switch*.

A food switch (also called a food swap) is a practical solution, especially for those of us who get overwhelmed by trying to make too many dietary changes at one time. The food switch breaks a big project—developing healthy eating habits—into smaller, more manageable bites.

Here's how it works. Let's say it's 8:00 p.m. and you're craving a sweet snack. That pint of ice cream in the freezer is calling your name. But what if you could find a snack that was lower in fat, sugar, and calories? Maybe some plain nonfat yogurt with fresh fruit blended in? Or a healthful smoothie with soy milk or almond milk as the base?

Here's another example. I know people who drink four to six cans of soda a day (or a combination of soda and energy drinks). I realize that it might not be realistic to "can" all those sodas on day one, so I challenge people to switch out just one of those sodas for the first week. "Go ahead with your three sodas," I tell them, "but replace the fourth one with some sparkling water and a bit of lemon, lime, or cranberry juice."

The following week, the goal escalates to two sodas and two flavored waters. Then it's on to one soda, two flavored waters, and one plain water. You can see where this is going, right? I have seen people give up their soda habit and eventually choose good old ice water as their go-to beverage.

By the way, you might be wondering why this example didn't mention diet soda as part of the swap. There's a good reason for that. A ten-year study of diet soda drinkers found that frequent diet soda or sugar-free soda imbibers were more likely to suffer a stroke or heart attack (or to die from some kind of cardiac-related illness) than people who didn't drink artificially sweetened beverages.[1]

If you're a potato chip or cheese puff aficionado, consider switching to whole-grain chips for a week. Then move on to air-popped popcorn or mixed nuts. I know some people who are now making their own apple, kale, or beet chips. This might never be you, but it shows just how far swapping and switching can go.

To make things even more interesting, challenge a friend or family member to do the switch with you. Make it an intrafamily competition, perhaps. Place a large jar or clear container in your kitchen. Every time someone switches junk food (or a junk beverage) for a healthier choice, put a quarter in the jar. At the end of the month, treat the family to a movie or some other outing.

Here is one example of a food switch.

Target Food: Ice Cream

- Week 1: Switch to low-fat ice cream with all-natural ingredients.
- Week 2: Switch to homemade frozen yogurt (or a small-batch variety from a health food store).
- Week 3: Switch to a yogurt parfait featuring plain Greek yogurt, fresh fruit, and a dash of vanilla extract.

I know a few people who have even started making their own ice cream by pureeing a few frozen bananas. Believe it or not, this one-ingredient ice cream is flavorful and has an appealing texture similar

---

[1] Candy Sagon, "Put Down the Diet Soda, Ladies. It's Bad for Your Heart," *AARP* (blog), April 2, 2014, http://blog.aarp.org/2014/04/02/put-down-the-diet-soda-ladies-its-bad-for-your-heart/.

to soft-serve ice cream. If you want to add a bit of flavor, you can toss in a pinch of salt, a little milk, and some fresh fruit.

You can do similar swaps with chips, bread, cookies, and so on. I encourage you to experiment, to be creative. I do this all the time. Make it an adventure, a quest. Eating healthfully should be fun.

> Make a careful exploration of who you are and the work you have been given, and then sink yourself into that. Don't be impressed with yourself. Don't compare yourself to others. Each of you must take responsibility for doing the creative best you can with your own life.
>
> GALATIANS 6:4–5 MSG

8

Don't Skip Breakfast

I get it—lots of people are too busy for breakfast. Many of us have to get ourselves ready for work *and* prepare the kids for their school day. Then we walk the dog, make sure the house or apartment is secure, and commute to work. And we'd like to do it all in time to beat the morning rush hour.

Yes, it can be tough to find the motivation to prepare a meal only to wolf it down so we can get everything done during our busy mornings.

But our moms and our health teachers were right about breakfast. When we wake up, we have been without nutrition for 12 hours or more. Breakfast provides an opportunity to literally break a fast. It's a chance to enjoy key nutrients that provide mental focus and the energy we need for the day ahead.

What's more, people who eat a good breakfast every day tend to make wiser food choices later in the day—and consume smaller meals in the evening. That's important because we tend to be less active in the evening. We are burning fewer calories.

I realize that many of us simply do not wake up hungry. But as with so many other things related to our health, we can train our bodies to be ready for breakfast.

If you've been a chronic breakfast skipper, you are probably not going to dive into a multicourse morning meal of pancakes, fresh eggs, ham or bacon, fresh fruit, fresh-squeezed juice, and a cup of brewed coffee.

That's okay. Start small—maybe a handful of almonds or peanuts. In a few days, add a serving of fresh fruit. Later, you can up your breakfast game to include a high-quality protein, like organic eggs or Greek yogurt. Eventually, you might find that your body will start craving a full morning meal.

I can't write a chapter about breakfast without hyping oatmeal a bit. Oatmeal is warm and filling. It's a complex carbohydrate with lots of soluble fiber. This makes it a cholesterol buster as well as a way to keep regular.

I should note here that those "quick oats" we see on the grocery store shelves have forfeited some of their fiber during processing. And some instant oatmeal has lots of added sugar, sugar you really don't need. So I recommend good old-fashioned rolled oats.

But the reigning champ in this category is steel-cut oatmeal. Yes, steel-cut oatmeal takes longer to cook, but it also takes longer to digest, making it a low-glycemic food. This means that steel-cut oatmeal is less likely to cause spikes in your blood sugar. (To save time, make a big batch of steel-cut oatmeal and refrigerate some of it. In the morning, microwave it, add a bit of milk and fresh fruit, and you are good to go.)

If you're convinced you're just never going to be a sit-down breakfast person, you can at least grab a hard-boiled egg or healthful granola bar to eat during your commute. Something is better than nothing.

One final note: When you shop the breakfast aisle of your favorite store, beware of the items that bill themselves as low fat or reduced fat. Often, these foods have had *beneficial* fats removed. I am talking about fats that boost satiety, which prevents or delays the midmorning hunger that often drives us to the vending machine or the box of donuts in the break room. Good fats also improve the absorption of antioxidants and fat-soluble vitamins, such as A, D, E, and K.

> Often, items billed as low fat, fat-free, or reduced fat have had *beneficial* fats removed. I am talking about fats that boost satiety, which prevents or delays the midmorning hunger that often drives us to the vending machine or the box of donuts in the break room.

Also, some low-fat, fat-free, or sugar-free foods are highly processed. They can contain fillers that have supplanted the fat. These fillers can be of questionable nutritional value. Often, fillers increase the carb content of a granola bar, for example, which negates the low-fat advantage.

Always opt for foods that are all natural rather than heavily processed. Remember, fat is not your true enemy. Poor quality and lots of chemicals and additives—those are what you should be fighting.

9

Stick to It!

I am including this chapter on perseverance in our diet and nutrition section, but I encourage you to use these principles as you exercise, train, reduce stress, and get more rest.

Our objective is to get healthier every day. That is a lofty goal, one that won't happen without focus, perseverance, and some support from friends, family, and health care professionals. And central to all these areas is changing your thinking—being transformed in your mind. Perseverance is a trait you can develop and strengthen.

I have certain bad habits that hinder my efforts to be as healthy as possible. Perhaps that is true for you as well. Here are a few habits I have identified—some from my own life and some from the lives of the people I train.

- not getting enough sleep
- stress eating (usually junk food)
- losing interest and motivation in an exercise program or diet
- smoking
- consuming too much alcohol
- spending too much time on hobbies that keep us sedentary for long periods of time (such as playing video games)

Do any of these sound familiar? Do they undermine your willpower? Please take a few minutes to think about a few habits that are not good for you. For example, do you often find yourself eating donuts, cake, and other sugar-laden treats that people bring to your workplace? That is a tough one for many of us. It's so easy to rationalize, "Hey, it's free food, so I might as well enjoy it. I'm saving money—that's a good thing, right?"

Or we might tell ourselves, "I know I shouldn't be eating these brownies, but I'll make up for it by eating something really healthful for dinner."

But when dinnertime comes around, it's all too easy to hit the fast-food drive-through on the way home. So no recompense for those brownies.

Here is a hard truth for all of us who want to live healthier: We must hold ourselves accountable. We need to accept that we all have bad habits, and when we start sliding back into them, we must be tough on ourselves. We must persevere.

It is important to note that long-term goals can sometimes be your enemy. Let me explain. Yes, big-picture goals are important, but it is so easy to get caught up in the weight-loss journey and use it as an excuse: "Yeah, I skipped breakfast today and had two donuts and a soda for lunch. But this is a marathon, not a sprint, right?"

The problem is that a marathon is run one step at a time, one mile at a time. What you do early in the race will affect the outcome.

As you strive to become a healthier person, you build success one day at a time. Celebrate your small daily victories—it takes perseverance to make those happen—and quickly "clean up" bad habits and run away from the temptations that hamstring your efforts.

> As you strive to become a healthier person, you build success one day at a time. Celebrate your small daily victories.

So please always start your meals with nutrient-rich foods that are loaded with vitamins, minerals, fiber, and healthy fats—especially omega-3 fatty acids, which have anti-inflammatory properties and can help lower your cholesterol level.

As a trainer and coach, I have been a crusader for omega-3-rich foods, like salmon, flax seeds, walnuts, and spinach. Foods like these pack essential fatty acids that your body needs. They will help you feel good on the inside and look great on the outside. Further, some promising new research indicates that walnuts might have a probiotic effect as well.

When you compare a lean filet of top-quality salmon with some packaged chemical cupcake…well, there really is no comparison. Junk food is empty calories and loads of chemicals and additives. Here is something I challenge people to do: Read the calorie content on that candy bar or sugary soda. Next, consider what nutrients you get with all those calories. Spoiler alert: Not many. Junk food is the epitome of empty calories.

Will that "snack cake" heal your muscles? Will it help you maintain a healthy weight? Does it provide nutrients your body needs? Does it even taste that great?

Before eating anything, ask yourself, "Is this a healthful food that will get me one step closer to my goals? And am I going to feel full of regret (and corn syrup and preservatives) later?"

Questions like these will prevent you from undermining what you have worked so hard to achieve. Let a candy bar be a very rare treat or a last resort.

So far we have looked at many don'ts with regard to sticking to a plan. Here are a couple of important dos.

First, embrace the power of protein. I could write a whole book on the power of lean and healthful protein. Protein helps your body produce vital hormones. It boosts your metabolism. It helps build and repair virtually every tissue in your body. If you are exercising (and you should be), you need protein.

As a bonus, protein does not spike your insulin levels like sugars and carbs can, so you will feel satiated longer. I try to include protein in every meal—lean meats, fish, eggs, and beans, like edamame, soybeans, pinto beans, white beans, kidney beans, and black beans.

When eating a meal, focus on your proteins first. Eat the protein before the fats and carbs. If you are going to fill up on one thing at mealtime, make it protein.

Also, consider the benefits of a cleanse or detox. Please do this under the direction of your doctor, trainer, or nutritionist because fad detox products abound. I favor making my own cleansing drink using real foods and tailoring a mixture to my specific needs.

I start with about six ounces of water. Then I add two tablespoons of apple cider vinegar that contains "mother of vinegar" (a beneficial combination of bacteria and acids). You're not going to get "the mother" in that big bargain gallon of white vinegar. I also like adding a dash or two of cayenne pepper. Cayenne is good for your digestive system, as is a bit of fresh lemon. I have found that these two ingredients are great for cleaning out my digestive tract.

If you have heard a lot of fuss about detoxing and wondered, "What's up with that?" here's the scoop: To lose weight and keep it off, you must ensure that your liver is operating at peak efficiency. Your liver is a three-pound miracle. It breaks down, eliminates, and neutralizes toxins. If your liver gets clogged with excess fats or toxins from junk food, it can't keep your body toxin-free. And you will not be able to burn fat at optimum efficiency.

For example, your body can handle a small amount of alcohol, consumed over a reasonable amount of time. When alcohol reaches your liver, it produces a toxic enzyme called acetaldehyde, which can damage liver cells and even cause permanent scarring if you drink too much.

Further, your liver needs water to do its job well. When alcohol enters the body, it acts as a diuretic. This forces the liver to pull water from other places in your body. This can lead to severe dehydration. That's why, if we overindulge, we're likely to wake up the next morning with a whopping headache.

This is a good time to point out why it is important to be detailed and specific when asking, "Do you drink?" If you mean chugging several beers in a short amount of time or doing shots, you are attacking your liver. If you sip a glass of red wine or two over the course of a healthy meal once in a while, that's another story. A better story.

Smoothie Stuff

Looking to make a healthy detoxing smoothie or just add more healthful foods to your diet? Consider these ingredients.

green leafy veggies
citrus fruits
broccoli sprouts
seeds and nuts, especially tree nuts
fresh garlic
onions
beans
green tea

10

Be Energy Efficient

Let's face it—it takes a lot of energy to lead a healthier lifestyle. In fact, it takes a lot of energy to live almost *any* kind of lifestyle. And many people try to get that energy in a can, in the form of energy drinks. The energy drink industry is projected to hit $84.8 billion by 2025.[1] For comparison, the athletic shoe industry was valued at $64.3 billion in 2017.[2]

You are probably familiar with the big names in the energy drink business. Most of them boast of their cutting-edge, trendy-sounding ingredients, but the real punch they pack comes from caffeine, which occurs naturally in coffee, tea, and cocoa. Caffeine, of course, is a stimulant. It accelerates blood circulation and helps your brain send messages more quickly. It can help you concentrate better, and it might even improve your reaction times.

When you down an energy drink, your heart pumps your blood faster and with more force. This effect, combined with that brain stimulation, boosts your energy.

So what's not to like, right? Well, let's take a closer look. Depending on the size of the product, an energy drink can deliver up to 242 milligrams of caffeine per serving. To put those 242 milligrams in perspective, consider that a 12-ounce can of cola or an 8-ounce cup of coffee contains about 50 milligrams of caffeine. (Of course, caffeine content varies from one style of coffee to the next. A double shot of espresso

---

[1] "Energy Drinks Market Size Worth $84.80 Billion by 2025," Grand View Research, July 2017, https:// www.grandviewresearch.com/press-release/global-energy-drinks-market.

[2] "Athletic Footwear Market Size, Share, & Trends," Grand View Research, April 2018, https://www .grandviewresearch.com/industry-analysis/athletic-footwear-market.

from your favorite coffee shop has about 150 milligrams, but that's still a lot less stimulation than you'll get from most energy drinks.)

Energy drink makers claim that their beverages are better than soda or coffee because they contain proprietary blends of herbs and other ingredients designed to provide a sustained energy boost—with no crash later on. However, this is a suspicious claim at best. I know a lot of people, including some athletes, who guzzle energy drinks like they are hooked on the stuff. If these beverages are truly crash-free, why do people need more and more energy infusions?

Further, especially among teens and tweens, there is concern about the side effects of energy drinks. These can include heart palpitations, chest pain, nervousness and anxiety, hot flashes, and blurred vision, just to name a few. To be fair, no solid independent research proves that energy drinks cause these maladies. But in 2013, the city of San Francisco sued one energy drink company, claiming it marketed its product to minors as young as six. (The drink company refuted the charge, and the outcome was pending at the writing of this book.)

All this said, do I sometimes use energy drinks? Yes. Do I shame clients who have an energy shot before a workout? No. But I also advise *everyone* to check with a doctor or nutritionist about this matter. Your health status and diet should be considered. And even then, I advise people to use an energy drink only occasionally. And no more than one beverage in one day.

An energy drink should be an occasional quick fix when better alternatives are not available. If you find yourself dragging in the middle of the afternoon workday, at the start of a workout, or on the last leg of a long car trip, just have a cup of coffee or tea instead.

> Develop smart lifestyle habits and strategies to keep yourself energized. Your energy doesn't have to come in a can.

And here is a much better way forward: Develop smart lifestyle habits and strategies to keep yourself energized. Your energy doesn't have to come in a can. Instead…

1. Eat three reasonably sized meals a day, augmented by a few healthy snacks spaced evenly during your day and night.
2. Drink lots of water. Keeping hydrated is foundational to good health anyway, and it helps digestion.
3. Exercise regularly.
4. Try to get a good night's sleep every night. (Emphasis on *try*. For some of us, this is a tough ask.)
5. When you are feeling tired, stressed, and cranky, instead of grabbing a can of liquid energy, practice relaxation techniques. Pray or meditate. Read or recite a favorite Scripture. Listen to a favorite inspirational artist.

I put energy drinks in the same category as candy bars and french fries. This is not the kind of stuff to make part of your regular diet; that would be unhealthy. But as an occasional indulgence or as a last resort, they are okay. Not great or even good—just okay.

But here is a problem I have observed, especially in the past five years or so. Even though energy drinks have not been proven to be physically addictive, they do become a habit, a psychological crutch, for many people. I know people who chug an energy drink before every workout. I know others whose sole breakfast item comes from a 20-ounce can.

It's worth repeating: An energy drink should be an occasional indulgence, not a staple. If you think you are becoming an addict, start tapering your weekly consumption. Use the food-swap technique I described earlier in chapter 7.

I try to keep my personal consumption at one or two cans a week. I encourage everyone I work with to be at least as stingy.

11

Make It Personal

As I have shared in this book, I have sometimes been unhappy with my weight—or my weight distribution. But in general, if I eat wisely and burn more calories than I eat, I shed fat, and my weight stays under control. However, one of my friends is in her midforties and is highly sensitive to many grains. She is not insulin resistant, but when she eats grains, her body revolts. Her stomach gets upset. You can hear it gurgling from across a room. She retains water, her mind fogs over, and she gains weight—even if she is working out faithfully.

Another friend, Rhonda, can't seem to gaze at a carb without adding a pound to her body weight. Rhonda is insulin resistant. This means her muscle cells don't allow insulin to bring in the carbs (which have been converted into glucose) to be stored as glycogen. And she needs that glycogen for energy. Her body tries to keep glucose from accumulating in the blood by diverting this sugar to her fat cells. These cells convert the glucose into even more fat.

So when Rhonda eats grains and starches—even just small portions—she gains weight in the form of fat. She can count calories all she wants; it doesn't help her lose weight.

I share these stories to emphasize that we are all unique. That's why each of us needs a custom-tailored diet and exercise regimen. We have different dietary challenges, so one solution doesn't work for everyone. That's why I encourage everyone to find doctors, nutritionists, and other professionals to "get personal" with you. Likewise, I urge you to modify and customize the advice you gain from books, including this one.

And let's take this personalization one step further. Our unique needs change as we get older or experience other life changes. For example, once we hit 45 or so, we tend to face challenges such as a lower carb threshold, insulin resistance, and emerging food sensitivities.

Case in point: I knew a guy who loved milk and ice cream and was able to consume both (in moderation) with no weight gain or digestive issues. Then when he hit 80, he became violently ill if he had even a couple of tablespoons of cream in his morning coffee. His doctor discovered he had developed a dairy allergy. And I don't mean just an allergy to lactose (milk sugar). His immune system now reacted negatively to the proteins in dairy, so he had to completely overhaul his diet.

However, some of the changes I am talking about can happen well before our AARP years. After age 30 or so, most of us simply can't burn carbs as efficiently as we did when we were younger. This means that the same diet that allowed us to be fit and trim at 25 will give us love handles and a paunch at 35.

> After age 30 or so, most of us simply can't burn carbs as efficiently as we did when we were younger. This means that the same diet that allowed us to be fit and trim at 25 will give us love handles and a paunch at 35.

Further, foods we could once handle with ease start causing inflammation and digestive issues. As women close in on menopause, their hormones are greatly influenced by grains and processed foods—stuff that once caused barely a blip on the digestive radar.

These factors can be disheartening, but they shouldn't be. A healthy lifestyle is not a one-and-done enterprise. It is an opportunity to keep fine-tuning and redesigning your lifestyle plan to make sure it's working for you.

I encourage you to keep embracing change. Look at each challenge that comes with aging as an opportunity to try new foods, new exercises, and new relaxation techniques. Each of us is unique, and each of us can find unique solutions to live better.

12

Do the Math

In this chapter, we're going to do a bit of math. You may not normally enjoy math, but I promise this won't be too painful. I also promise you can use this in everyday life.

Let's start with a few average calorie counts for common foods.

- A slice of whole-wheat bread has about 70 calories.
- A glazed donut has about 250 calories.
- A 12-ounce can of (nondiet) soda has about 150 calories.
- A 1-ounce serving of caramels contains about 115 calories.
- A light beer (12 ounces) has about 95 calories.
- A regular beer (12 ounces) has about 150 calories.
- A 3-ounce steak has 240 calories. (And I know—3 ounces is not much of a steak!)
- An unpeeled apple has about 125 calories.
- A banana has about 105 calories.

With these numbers in mind, consider that each pound of stored fat in our bodies represents approximately 3,550 calories. Simple math tells us that we need to expend more calories than we absorb if we want to lose weight. So to lose just one pound of fat, you need to spend about 3,550 more calories than you are taking in from your foods and beverages.

Most of us Americans consume about 3,000 calories a day. But how many calories do we burn? Of course, the totals vary widely depending on your age, weight, activity level, and so on, but it is estimated that if you did virtually nothing all day, you would burn about 1,400 calories just maintaining your basic bodily functions. Sitting and doing absolutely nothing burns about 75 calories an hour. If you read during that hour, you burn about 112 calories an hour. (Just by reading this book, you're shredding an extra 37 calories an hour. You're welcome!)

According to choosemyplate.gov (formerly MyPyramid.gov), a 30-year-old man who is active for 30 to 60 minutes a day burns about 2,800 calories daily.[1] I bet you are already way ahead of me on the math. Even the average young and somewhat-active man doesn't burn as many calories as he is taking in (2,800 versus 3,000). And when you consider that many people consume more than 4,000 calories daily, it's no wonder that too many Americans are gaining weight.

Here is the challenge faced by those of us striving to lose weight. To shed just one pound of fat a week, you need an average daily deficit of about 500 calories. To arrive at this deficit, the choice is simple: Exercise an extra 500 calories' worth or consume 500 fewer calories—every single day. Using the calorie totals from the beginning of this chapter, this would mean (roughly speaking) cutting one can of soda, one can of light beer, a steak, and a banana from your daily meals and snacks. What if you don't drink light beer? Well, say goodbye to one *more* banana.

I know that all this "food math" can be a little depressing—just like regular math for some of us. But I want to make an important point. I encourage you to think of food as fuel for your life, as a source of key nutrients. And I also believe that meals with family and friends can be sacred times—times of laughter, sharing, praying, bonding, gratefulness, fellowship, and faith.

I'm a huge advocate of family mealtime. Or friends mealtime.

What's more, skipping meals and starving yourself of the nutrition you need to continue functioning at an optimal level is not a smart way to lose weight. This is why so many people fail when they try "extreme diets."

---

[1] USDA, ChooseMyPlate.gov, "Get Your MyPlate Plan," www.choosemyplate.gov/MyPlatePlan. Input your information on this site to get specific results.

Now, let's find out what happens when we add exercise to the equation. *Runner's World* magazine has a great "Calories Burned Running Calculator" on its website.[2] You can input your weight, distance run, and running time and discover how many calories you burned on a run. I have a distance-running friend named Tom. Let's use him as an example. On Tom's most recent 7.5-mile run, he burned almost 1,200 calories. That's more than twice the daily deficit target of 500 calories.

I realize not everyone is likely to run 7.5 miles in a single effort, but I hope this gives you an idea of how exercise can contribute to weight loss and weight maintenance.

I want to emphasize that Tom doesn't run 7.5 miles every day, even though running is a staple of his exercise program. Few people amass that kind of mileage. But the good news is that at Tom's weight and running pace, he needs to run only 3 miles a day to burn about 500 calories. In fact, he can walk (briskly) 3 miles a day and get about the same total. I can walk and get about the same total. (I am almost the same age as Tom and only about 10 or 15 pounds heavier.) The only difference is that it takes me about 24 minutes to run 3 miles, while walking that same distance takes about 50 minutes. A lot of people don't realize that walking and running burn almost the same number of calories per mile. The only difference is the time it takes.

> A lot of people don't realize that walking and running burn almost the same number of calories per mile. The only difference is the time it takes.

If distance running isn't your thing (it isn't mine either), I have good news for you. An hour of bicycling burns about 650 calories an hour. An hour of tennis? About 420. If you precede or follow your aerobic efforts with some weight lifting or resistance training, that will burn another 265 calories per hour.

---

[2] "Calories Burned Running Calculator," *Runner's World*, June 22, 2018, https://www.runnersworld.com/training/a20801301/calories-burned-running-calculator/.

It's important to keep in mind that exercise might increase your appetite, so I encourage you to keep an eye on what you are eating. If you want to lose some weight, maintain your calorie intake while increasing your activity level.

Some people experience a dent in their appetite when they start working out as their bodies adjust to the new regimen. This might seem like a welcome change, but remember to avoid restricting your food intake too much. If your body thinks it's starving, your brain will dial down your resting metabolic rate. This will make it even harder to achieve that calorie deficit you are striving for.

As a personal trainer, I encourage my clients to set a weight-loss goal of a half pound a week. That might not seem like much of a goal, but this is a process, a lifestyle change. And it's manageable. With this as your target, you need to achieve an average daily calorie deficit of 250. I have seen person after person achieve this goal by making a small but targeted reduction in junk foods and sugary beverages—combined with a reasonable increase in exercise or general daily activity.

Keep in mind that a half pound of fat loss per week will get you a 26-pound weight loss in one year. In two years, you will have lost 52 pounds. In three years, 78 pounds. That's the kind of math anyone can love.

And because this approach is so doable, you can keep it up for as long as you need to. If you have gained some weight over the past few years, you probably didn't gain it at the rate of a pound a week. That would yield a weight gain of 52 pounds in a single year. Most likely, you gained weight at a slower rate—possibly due to some change in your life. Many of the people I train or coach tell me a similar story: "I was relatively fit and healthy until…

I had my first child.

I got married.

I got a desk job.

I hurt my knee playing tennis.

I turned 50."

So I recommend you lose weight the same way—one day and one step at a time.

The next time someone promises you can lose a pound or more a week, do the math and remind yourself that patience and perseverance are more than wonderful virtues. They actually work for you.

13

Value Your Body as a Work of Art

As an athlete, coach, trainer, and human being, I'm constantly amazed at the design of the human body. Consider a few of the ways God made you and me to live and thrive.

Your Brain

- Your brain represents about 2 percent of your body weight, but it uses 20 percent of your total oxygen and calorie intake.[1]

- Your brain has approximately 86 billion neurons.[2] One piece of brain tissue the size of a grain of sand has 100,000 neurons and one billion synapses that all communicate with one another.[3]

- There are about 400 miles of blood vessels in your brain.[4]

- Your brain's storage capacity is around a million gigabytes. In DVR terms, that's enough to hold 3 million hours of movies and TV shows.[5]

---

[1] Marcus Paichle and Debra Gusnard, "Appraising the Brain's Energy Budget," *Proceedings of the National Academy of Sciences of the United States of America*, August 6, 2002, http://www.pnas.org/content/99/16/10237.full.

[2] Bradley Voytek, "Brain Metrics," *Scitable* (blog), May 20, 2013, https://www.nature.com/scitable/blog/brain-metrics/are_there_really_as_many.

[3] Daniel Amen, "The Incredible Brain!," Solution Resources EAP, http://www.solutionresources.net/The_Incredible_Brain_-D_Amen-.pdf.

[4] Marilyn Cipolla, "Anatomy and Ultrastructure," in *The Cerebral Circulation* (San Rafael, CA: Morgan & Claypool Life Sciences, 2009), ch. 2, https://www.ncbi.nlm.nih.gov/books/NBK53086/.

[5] Paul Reber, "What Is the Memory Capacity of the Human Brain?," *Scientific American*, May 1, 2010, https://www.scientificamerican.com/article/what-is-the-memory-capacity/.

Your Heart

- Your heart beats about 100,000 times a day, 35 million times a year, and more than 2.5 billion times in an average lifetime.[6]

- The heart has its own electrical supply and can continue to beat even when it's separated from the body.[7]

- Each minute, your heart pumps 1.5 gallons of blood.[8] In one day, the blood travels a total of 12,000 miles, or the equivalent of traveling coast to coast across the United States four times.[9]

Your Cells

- You have more than 37 trillion cells in your body, give or take a few thousand.[10]

- Cells range in size from about 7 to 300 micrometers. (To put this in perspective, the dot on this "i" is about 100 micrometers wide.)[11]

- Each cell in your body contains your genetic code, or DNA. Your code is unique to you. It directs the cellular activity needed for your structure and function.[12]

- Cells self-destruct if they become damaged or undergo infection. This is your body's natural defense against disease.[13]

---

[6] "Amazing Heart Facts," Nova, http://www.pbs.org/wgbh/nova/eheart/facts.html.

[7] "Health Essentials," Cleveland Clinic, October 4, 2017, https://health.clevelandclinic.org/2016/08/2 2-amazing-facts-about-your-heart-infographic/.

[8] "Health Essentials."

[9] "Amazing Heart Facts."

[10] Eva Bianconi et al., "An Estimation of the Number of Cells in the Human Body," *Annals of Human Biology* 40, no. 6 (2013), http://www.tandfonline.com/doi/abs/10.3109/03014460.2013.807878.

[11] John Berardi et al., *The Essentials of Sport and Exercise Nutrition* (Toronto, Canada: Precision Nutrition, 2016), 41.

[12] John Berardi et al., *The Essentials of Sport and Exercise Nutrition*, 43.

[13] Regina Bailey, "10 Facts About Cells," ThoughtCo, March 9, 2018, https://www.thoughtco.com/facts-about-cells-373372.

Your Bones and Muscles

Muscles make up more than half your body weight.
There are about 696 muscles in your body
(give or take a muscle or two).

- The adult human body has 206 bones. Twenty-six of these are found in the foot, and 54 are found in the hand and wrist.[14]

- Bone is living tissue that constantly replenishes itself. Every seven years, you have a brand-new skeleton.[15]

- Muscles make up more than half your body weight. There are approximately 696 muscles in your body.[16]

- The busiest muscles in your body are your eye muscles. They move more than 100,000 times a day.[17] The next time you are thinking, "My eyes are tired," contemplate this fact!

Are you starting to get the picture? This is just a small fraction of the amazing facts about your body's design. And there are hundreds more that I don't have room to include. Things like your unique genetic characteristics—your hair and eye color, skin type, voice, and so much more. Considering these amazing truths helps me appreciate my God-given body more—and inspires me to take better care of it. I hope the same for you.

---

[14] "Fun Facts About Bones and Joints," Beth Israel Deaconess Medical Center, March 1, 2011, https://www.bidmc.org/about-bidmc/blogs/wellness-insight-landing/bones-and-joints/fun-facts-about-bones-and-joints.

[15] Kim Stearns, "13 Strange and Interesting Facts About Your Bones," Cleveland Clinic, October 26, 2015, https://health.clevelandclinic.org/2015/10/13-strange-interesting-facts-bones-infographic/.

[16] Marsha Clarke, "The Muscular System: Did You Know…," *Marsha G. Clarke RMT* (blog), http://marshaclarkermt.com/10-fun-facts-on-the-muscular-system/.

[17] Clarke, "The Muscular System."

14

Don't Think Fat

met my wife (now my ex-wife) when I was in the air force and stationed at Misawa Air Base in Japan. She was a marine. The guys in the marines had been "stealing" my female air force colleagues, so I figured turnabout was fair play. (I was 20 at the time and not very mature. Obviously.) Anyway, I met this young woman, and we were married within a few months.

Before long, she decided it was time for me to meet her parents. They came from Chicago to Japan to visit us. I liked them immediately. A lot of people think "Midwest" when they think of Chicago, but I find that people from Chicago have more of a Boston or New York vibe to them—confident, no nonsense. My new in-laws were fun to be around.

However, one thing disturbed me. From the time they woke up until they were ready to call it a night, they made food the center of almost every conversation. They didn't eat just to fuel their bodies; they ate because they *loved* to eat. I had never encountered people who enjoyed food so much.

I heard questions like this at least 20 times a day: "What do you have a taste for? What sounds good to eat right now?"

As you might guess, my new in-laws were both overweight, and I knew my bride would probably follow suit someday. When she was with her parents, she ate like they did. And she told me that after her military service overseas was complete, she wanted to live as close as possible to her parents. She didn't view them as a cautionary tale; she wanted to be just like them.

Even back then, I knew this would not be good for her health. You might have heard the saying "You are who you roll with." That is true in so many ways. And when it comes to being healthy, it's so important to have at least some friends and family members who share your goals and values. People who think the way you do, who inspire you to be your best.

Of course, this isn't always possible. We don't get to choose our neighbors, coworkers, or most of our relatives. Sometimes even our friends are chosen for us. But when you find yourself regularly in the company of people who don't live healthfully, you must think differently and act differently than they do. If you follow the same bad habits as those around you, how can you expect to look and feel healthier than they do?

Often, people who live unhealthy lifestyles are less than honest with themselves and with those around them. When it comes to things like exercise and diet, they coddle themselves and others.

I encourage you to foster relationships with people who challenge you physically, mentally, and spiritually. Seek out honest relationships, even if that means you have to change your thinking. Even if it means getting an occasional kick in the butt.

I am thankful for friends who have told me, "Do you want to look better? Then do something about it!" or "Do you really think you can eat that many sweets and avoid getting fat?"

Let's face it. Most of us are always doing at least a few things we know we shouldn't be doing, whether it's downing too many beers on the weekend or trying to survive on meager sleep week after week. We need people in our lives who will call us out. Not because they are mean or judgmental but because they care.

> Time and again, I have seen how things like a strong
> relationship with God and a great support system—
> family friends, work colleagues—make a huge
> difference in a person's health.

My life experiences have taught me that living a long, healthy, and meaningful life means building strong connections between our physical bodies and our mental, emotional, and spiritual well-being. A good life is more than the absence of disease or infirmity. In fact, I have worked with people who had physical disabilities but were much healthier than others with no significant physical challenges. Time and again, I have seen how things like a strong relationship with God and a great support system—family, friends, work colleagues—make a huge difference in a person's health.

This book has three parts, but I often mention spirituality in the diet and nutrition section or talk about nutrition in chapters about stress management and rest. This is intentional. Good health is about balance. It's a multifaceted quest. It's a life-enriching quest. My hope and prayer is that this book will make that balancing act effective and rewarding for you.

15

Crack the Cheat Code

I wish that whoever came up with the concept of dietary "cheat days" had chosen his or her words more carefully. The word "cheat" packs lots of baggage, and it brings lots of guilt and confusion to the table—literally. The whole idea of rewarding yourself with a cheat day creates a Gordian knot of emotions and confusion.

Unfortunately, the term is here to stay. We have to deal with it. Here's how I deal with it: There are no cheat days. Enjoying a rare indulgence beyond our normal diet isn't a failure or a transgression. I wish cheat days were called "reward days" or "special indulgence days."

> Here's how I deal with cheat days: There are no cheat days. Enjoying a rare indulgence beyond our normal diet isn't a failure or a transgression. I wish cheat days were called "reward days" or "special indulgence days."

When I eat a so-called cheat food, I enjoy it to the fullest. I enjoy the experience. I enjoy the chance to reward myself for a week of great workouts and smart eating. I feel good, not guilty. I feel thankful that God has provided so many delicious things to eat in this world. I encourage the people I train to do the same. In fact, I don't allow them to use the term "cheat food" or "cheat day" unless they can use those terms with zero guilt. After all, what reasonable person plans to do something that will induce guilt?

If you're eating something, you should be able to do it with gratitude in your heart and a smile on your face. The way you feel about the food you eat might be just as important as the food itself. Did you know that if you eat a donut and feel disgusted as a result, your body releases the same stress chemicals as when you yearn for a donut but deprive yourself of it?

So the trick is to eat that donut (or cheat food of your choice) and feel no guilt. If you can cross this mental barrier, you will find that eating a donut—or not eating it—becomes no big deal. That donut no longer presents a titanic test of your willpower. It's just some dough and maybe some frosting that you enjoy occasionally. Or something you can skip in favor of a banana or a carrot. Just because you want to. I tell people all the time, "If we are stuck with this 'cheat day' terminology, then we should be able to cheat on our cheat days, right?"

I don't have to consume the hot-fudge sundae just because I thought about it earlier. I can have plain ice cream or sorbet—or nothing at all. I am in control. That's the key to cracking the cheat code.

I strongly encourage you to crack your own personal cheat code. Change your thought patterns if you need to. Change the way you talk to yourself. It's not about giving yourself blanket permission to eat sugary foods any time you feel you deserve them; it's about asking yourself, "I know that I might deserve a donut today because of how well I have done this week, but do I really want that donut? Is it going to provide the fuel I need today? Is it really the best way to reward myself right now?"

You will occasionally drive by an ice cream shop and imagine how good a sundae would taste. Or someone at work is going to bring in some delicious homemade cookies, and your mouth will start watering. You're probably going to eat a cookie. So eat it with appreciation and enjoyment, not guilt. If you have to take a walk on your break to feel less guilty, then do that. If you need to skip dessert after dinner that night, skip away.

In short, treat your body and your mind as if they belong to someone you love. Because in fact, they do.

16

Understand the 70/30 Principle

If you've done a lot of reading on the topic of health, you have probably heard of the 70/30 principle, which should be more accurately called the 70/30 generalization. It's one of those classic good news–bad news situations. The bad news is that about 30 percent of our health and vitality are determined by our genetics, our age, and our gender. The good news is that the lion's share of our health is in our hands. About 70 percent of living healthfully is determined by lifestyle choices, not genetics.

For example, breast cancer is a major health concern for women. Many of us have seen a close friend or relative die too young because of this disease. However, contrast the approximately 40,000 American women who die of breast cancer every year with the 500,000 women who die from conditions that are largely preventable. Specifically, I am referring to high blood pressure and coronary artery disease, which includes things like heart attack, stroke, and congestive heart failure.

To put things in even sharper perspective, for each woman who dies from breast cancer, more than two die from stroke, and almost nine die from a heart attack.

When someone tells me, "I'm doomed when it comes to health. I come from a bad gene pool," here is my response: "Avoid added sugar in your diet. Focus on a moderate intake of healthy fats. Eat lots of fruits and vegetables. You will live longer. You will lower your risk of diabetes and cardiovascular disease as well as obesity, cognitive impairment, and dementia. Your genes are not your destiny."

Like me, you probably have a genetic risk for certain diseases or metabolic challenges. That can make you feel as if you're beginning a race way behind the starting line, but keep in mind that you probably also have a few genetic gifts, courtesy of your ancestors.

And please remember that the overwhelming percentage of health factors is under your control. In fact, some trainers and doctors I know say that the 70/30 principle should be called the 80/20 principle.

Lifestyle trumps genetics. We can make our lives so much better if we eat right, exercise regularly, deal effectively with stress, and get enough sleep and downtime. There is so much we can do to live longer and live better.

I encourage you to keep the 70/30 principle at the forefront of your mind. It will help you in so many ways. For example, I have some friends who don't watch what they eat and exercise sporadically. "It's okay," they tell me, "I have good genes."

I tell them, "You can have the best genetic makeup in the world, but if you don't take good care of yourself, you will age quicker than you should. And you might fall victim to heart disease, obesity, or something else that is preventable."

And of all the lifestyle choices you can make, food has the biggest impact. This might seem counterintuitive. We all seem to know a person who has a terrible diet but seems to stay in good shape by exercising religiously. But as you will read in part 2, you simply cannot out-train a bad diet.

You can't out-train a bad diet.

Eventually, all those bad dietary choices will catch up with you. While doing research for this book, I was amazed at the number of books with titles like *Food Is Medicine* or *Food as Medicine* or *Food Is Better Than Medicine*. More and more doctors and nutritionists are reminding their patients and clients that food should do more than provide our bodies with the energy we need to get through each day. Food should nurture and maintain our health.

God designed the human body to build new blood cells, skin cells, muscle, and bone. As we learned in chapter 13, we have a vast communication system that constantly monitors messages and warnings—and makes course corrections when necessary. But we need to care for our bodies so all these complex systems keep working. You can't put corn syrup in your car's gas tank or crankcase and expect it to perform well.

Our bodies are constantly regenerating. We shed dead skin cells by the hour and replace them with fresh new cells. A similar change is happening to your bones and muscles—right now. And the quality of all those cells in your body depends heavily on the quality of the building materials you supply your body, meal after meal, snack after snack. "You are what you eat" is more than a cliché. It's the truth.

> "You are what you eat" is more than a cliché. It's the truth.

The years ahead of you can be your best years. And you don't have to give up all the foods you love and consume nothing but kombucha and kale chips for the rest of your life. But I do encourage you to keep the 70/30 ratio in mind so that you will eat and drink more thoughtfully. All those books are right: Food is medicine. Sometimes it's long-term, preventive medicine. And in some cases, people can experience almost immediate improvement by eliminating junk food and junk beverages from their diets.

Your food and beverage choices are rarely neutral. They can make your life so much better or so much worse. Thinking 70/30 will help you make better choices. I am 100 percent sure of that.

17

Water: Way More Than Another Beverage

Water. It's all around us. It's in us. In a way, it *is* us. The human body is about two-thirds water, and water affects every bodily function in one way or another. In fact, I am sometimes asked, "What is the one thing a person can do to improve his or her health right now?" My go-to response is, "Drink more water."

> I am sometimes asked, "What is the one thing a person can do to improve his or her health right now?" My go-to response is, "Drink more water."

I could probably write a whole book extolling the virtues of water, but instead, let's look at a few of its best benefits.

Water Can Help You Lose Weight

If you are trying to manage your weight or simply avoid the occasional episodes of overeating, drink a glass of water before your meals. At a restaurant, I always ask for water first. I make sure I down a glass before I even decide what to eat. And at home, I never sit down to a meal without my H_2O.

That premeal beverage helps us eat less by making us feel full. And being well hydrated aids your body's digestive process. By the way, I have found that many people mistake midmorning or midafternoon hunger for thirst. It's one way that weight gain can sneak up on us. The next time you feel fatigued or sluggish, especially between meal times, sip a glass of clear, cold water instead of grabbing a sugary or salty snack. You might find that water is just what you need to perk you up.

It Keeps You Cool When Your Workouts Get Hot

Within reason, it's okay to go for a run or bike ride on a hot day—but only if you are properly hydrated. The hotter the workout, the more you sweat, and you need to replace those lost fluids. If you are a marathoner or long-haul cyclist, you might need a sports drink fortified with electrolytes and carbs. But for many people, a trusty bottle of water will help you avoid dehydration during that tennis match or power walk. Even if you are just doing a short workout on a hot day, maintaining your fluid balance is important. So drink up. You might find that your performance is better—and that you are less fatigued afterward.

It Keeps You Going...

...if you know what I mean. Water keeps you regular by helping dissolve fats and soluble fiber. Drinking water is one of the best ways to avoid constipation. Moreover, it lessens the burden on your kidneys and liver by helping flush waste products from your system.

Without going into too much graphic detail here, water binds with fiber to make elimination faster and easier. When you don't drink enough water and other fluids, your colon will pull water from your stools. That, in turn, increases your risk of constipation. And that's all we need to say about *that*.

It Might Protect You Against Some Forms of Cancer

There is some promising early research indicating that the greater the fluid intake, the lower the incidence of bladder cancer. And the most promising results have come when that fluid is water. It's too early to make concrete cause-and-effect conclusions, but it stands to reason that water helps you urinate more frequently, thereby preventing the buildup of carcinogens in your bladder. Staying hydrated may also reduce your risk of colon cancer and breast cancer.

I want to emphasize that more research is needed, but the logic seems clear. And considering water's other benefits, this is just one more good reason to increase your intake.

It's a Natural Headache Remedy

Are you one of those people who gets a headache if you get dehydrated? Me too. Further, dehydration has long been identified as a trigger for migraines. The good news is that a glass of water or two can often provide total relief for some headache sufferers. I tell all my headache-prone friends and clients to stay hydrated throughout the day, especially days that are physically or emotionally challenging.

And if you are a migraine sufferer like me, be sure to drink water along with whatever medication you might be taking. I recommend drinking two to four cups of water as soon as you feel a headache coming on. Often, this will help you feel much better in an hour or so, even if you don't take any medication.

It's Good for Your Kidneys

I touched on this earlier. Our kidneys remove waste from our bodies, they help control our blood pressure, and they keep our fluid levels in balance. And a kidney can't work all this magic without enough water to keep it functioning properly.

It's an All-Natural Energy Drink

Next time you feel as if you're ready to bonk during a workout or even before one, try drinking some water. Feeling tired is one of the first signs of dehydration. (By the way, dehydration can also impair your mental focus, memory, and motor skills.) Filling up with some H_2O could give you just the boost you need.

I know that some of us like a little fizz and flavor in our workout beverages. So how about adding a couple of lemon or lime slices to some sparkling water? Or a splash of fruit juice? This is a much better choice than a sugary soda or any drink laden with artificial sweeteners and chemicals.

It Protects Our Joints and Cartilage

Water helps keep the cartilage around our joints hydrated and subtle. It's like lubrication for the joints. Water also protects our spinal cords and bodily tissues, keeping us healthy from the inside out. Remember when I said water *is* us? That's especially true when it comes to cartilage, that miraculous rubbery material that connects our bones, allows our joints to function, acts as a shock absorber, and more. Cartilage is about 85 percent water, so we must be hydrated to keep this vital material healthy.

This chapter took a while to write. I need a glass of water now. How about you?

18

Keep a Running List of Rules

As a military veteran, I can appreciate the importance of rules for keeping life in order and clarifying procedures and processes. Whatever your goals are, it's great to have a list of guidelines to refer to so you are not flying by the seat of your pants all the time.

In my quest to be at my healthiest, I have created a list of rules. These are the most important things I want and need to remember about nutrition, exercise, rest, recovery, and so on.

The list below is from several years ago. I often make changes—categorizing, rewording, adding new information, and so on. I encourage you to do something similar and see if it helps you. I know it has helped me and many of the people I train. Whether you keep your list in a notebook, on your phone or iPad, or on a whiteboard in your house, you might find that it helps to have things in print.

> Your list of rules should support your goals. And they should help you avoid your blind spots or temptations.

Your rules should support your goals. And they should help you avoid your blind spots or temptations. As you will surmise from this early list, I started writing things based on what was going on in my life at the time—my priorities and pitfalls.

Matt Dragon's Running List of Rules

Eat lean meat at every meal if possible.

Eat beans often. (Healthful beans, not pork and beans drenched in a sugary sauce.)

Avoid sugar and avoid bread as much as possible.

Eat lots of fruits and vegetables.

Meats and veggies sautéed in olive oil = good. Meats and veggies breaded and deep-fried = not so much.

Focus on good fats—coconut oil, macadamia nut oil, butter, olive oil, grapeseed oil, tree nuts, and so on.

Berries and plain yogurt taste amazing, and they are amazing for me!

When in doubt, have another glass of water. Drink water even when not in doubt.

Limit calories from fruit juice.

When drinking beer, remember, "Not too much, not too often."

When drinking wine, see above.

Have the occasional candy bar. "Occasional" is the operative word.

Weight train to build muscle.

Play a sport!

Start taking zinc to build the immune system and fight free radicals.

Start taking magnesium to help regulate muscle and nerve functions.

Make sure to get enough iodine.

Get at least one hour of fresh air and sunlight every day.

Every morning, drink a big glass of water before doing light calisthenics.

Drink (more!) water with honey, cinnamon, and fresh lemon juice every day before breakfast.

Drink mint tea with fresh ginger several times a week, especially before bedtime.

Reduce stress as much as possible.

Try to learn something new every day by reading and by doing.

After a hard workout day, take a day off—but no more than
    one day.

No cell phone while training!

Try to get eight or nine hours of sleep every night.

I hope my list gives you some ideas. Your list will probably grow and become better organized. But the cool thing is that these rules start to become part of your DNA. Some things, like drinking water first thing in the morning, are now such a part of my routine and so important to my overall well-being, I would do them even if I lost my list. It's like putting on my shoes before I go outside or locking the door before I head to work.

19

Mind the Labels

So much of your success in eating healthfully depends on selecting the best foods when you shop. Food labels offer a wealth of information if you know how to digest them properly. As you strive to make the best choices for you and your family, focus on the list of ingredients and nutritional information. Ignore the hype words, like "all natural," "low-fat," or "fat-free." (I roll my eyes anytime I see a box of candy labeled "fat-free." Yes, those little cylinders of sugar and gelatin have no fat, but that doesn't make them health food.)

You don't need to be a scientist or nutritionist to shop healthy and eat healthy. You just need to be vigilant. Here are a few hints.

Check the Serving Size

As you count calories, fat grams, and the like, note the serving size. For example, you might think a "personal size" cherry pie is a great snack. After all, it's rather small compared to a regular pie, and it has fruit in it. But be careful. It might offer "only" 20 fat grams, for example, just one-fourth of your daily recommended total. But is it 20 fat grams per serving? And according to the label, how many servings does that mini pie offer? Three? Seriously? So just how much fat does this little pastry *truly* pack? Sixty fat grams! I think I'll pass.

Beware of Hidden Sugars

High-calorie, nutritionally bankrupt sugars, like high-fructose corn syrup, lurk everywhere. Why? They're cheap and sweet, so they make things taste good. Don't eat any more of this goo than you must. Before you buy ketchup, steak sauce, barbecue sauce, pizza sauce, peanut butter, tomato sauce—virtually anything—check the ingredients. You'll be surprised how many products include high-fructose corn syrup as a primary ingredient—if not the number one ingredient. (I'm looking at you, beef sticks.) Avoid them if you can. After all, you wouldn't pour syrup on your steak or your pizza, would you? (By the way, most people know that corn syrup is synonymous with sugar, but beware of other euphemisms, such as malt syrup, cane syrup, invert syrup, fructose, and maltodextrin.)

> High-calorie, nutritionally bankrupt sugars, like high-fructose corn syrup, lurk everywhere. Why? They're cheap and sweet, so they make things taste good. Don't eat any more of this goo than you must.

Watch for Deceptive Labels

Make sure you're getting what you want, not a sugary substitute. If you want 100 percent pure fruit juice, watch for terminology like cranberry juice *cocktail* or fruit juice *drink*. These are synonyms for syrupy, artificially flavored water with a few dribbles of actual fruit juice mixed in—just enough to warrant using "juice" on the label and not getting smacked down by the FDA.

By the way, you should be just as diligent with fast foods. I recently visited a fast-food establishment, and I decided to read the ingredients on a packet of honey sauce. It was the word "sauce" that caught my eye. Here are the ingredients: high fructose corn syrup, sugar, corn syrup, honey, caramel color.

Yes, you read that correctly. Honey was the *fourth* ingredient in the honey sauce! The first three ingredients were cheap, ultrasweet, processed sugars.

Don't be fooled by appearances and reputation. Everyone knows that tuna salad sandwiches are good for you, right? Loaded with omega-3s. Besides, "salad" is right there in the name! So if the lunch choice came down to tuna versus roast beef (ugh—red meat), determining which is healthier is a no-brainer, isn't it? Not so much. A tuna salad sandwich made with mayo packs 680 calories and 40.5 grams of fat, while a roast beef sandwich (also with mayo) carries 382 calories and 16.9 grams of fat.

Resources

To get the nutritional lowdown on your favorite foods, visit websites like calorieking.com and livestrong.com. And for a great smackdown comparison on various fast-food and chain restaurant entrées, check out eatthis.com or read the books in the "Eat This, Not That" series from Rodale Press.

For even more information on eating right (and being label smart), check out these resources.

- www.choosemyplate.gov
- www.health.gov/dietaryguidelines
- www.nlm.nih.gov/medlineplus
- www.myrecipes.com/recipe-finder

Supplements

My advice on minding food labels also applies to other items you might encounter at your local grocery store, like supplements, including minerals, herbs, botanicals, enzymes, and amino acids. I encourage caution when it comes to these pills, capsules, tablets, tinctures, and so on. I understand the desire to supplement our diets with extra boosts. However, we should opt for supplements that are safe, effective, and backed by solid research.

As you might know, the supplements on the shelves of your local drugstores and grocery stores are not regulated in the United States, and there are so many brands and varieties that it is difficult to know exactly what you are getting.

You will probably see boasts like "clinically proven" or "backed by research" on a supplement's packaging, but that research was probably done by the same people who package and sell the product. Check with a doctor or nutritionist. He or she might be aware of some less biased research conducted independently.

Finally—and I say this as a person who takes only one prescription—there are many pharmaceutical drugs that are inexpensive and have been proven to be safe and effective for various conditions. (I know that certain medications make the news when their prices skyrocket, but that is often the exception, not the rule.)

For example, I am all for any supplement that might help people control their cholesterol levels or combat hypertension. But there are prescription medications proven to address these challenges. These medications have undergone a rigorous approval process, and many of them have a multiyear track record to support them. What's more, many of them are very affordable under most health insurance plans. I have friends and family who spend about $12 per month on statins (for heart health). You would be hard-pressed to find any herbal supplement that is so affordable.

Let's say you have read about zuzi extract. (Yes, I am making this up. Please don't head for the grocery store on a zuzi quest.) When shopping, you need to look for the specific name of the zuzi plant and its species. What part of the plant has been suggested or proven to be effective? The root, the leaf, the flower, the bark? Maybe it was a combination of these.

Is the powder in those capsules made of the whole plant or merely dried leaves from the plant? Or is it an extract from the root? The stems? And what difference do all these variables mean for your health?

Confused yet? Consider this: You also need to know what percentage of your zuzi capsules is standardized. A standardized herbal extract, for example, has its components present in a specific and guaranteed amount from capsule to capsule. This means that those zuzi benefits are consistent from one batch to the next.

By the way, the supplements made from a whole plant or even plant parts are not standardized the same way extracts are. That's right, when it comes to supplements, even the standardizations themselves are not standardized! That's why some doctors recommend specific brands of supplements—and even specific varieties of those brands.

Here's the bottom line: I wouldn't take any supplement without specific advice from a doctor or nutritionist. And even then I would ask for regular blood tests (or some other diagnostic measure) to evaluate whether a supplement is doing what it's supposed to. I recommend the same for you.

20

Know Your Trouble Foods

Do you have friends or relatives who have allergies or other sensitivities to various foods? Have you ever wondered if you might have some unknown trouble foods?

I have seen people make huge health breakthroughs when they pinpointed a troublesome food or beverage—and then eliminated it. Sometimes this is permanent. But sometimes a food can be removed from the menu and then reintroduced slowly and strategically, based on how one's body responds.

Unfortunately, most people have no idea they have a sensitivity to certain foods. They have symptoms, but they blame them on stress, the aging process, or allergies to something other than food. So they soldier on, having almost forgotten what it's like to feel good. They have no idea that simply removing a few foods and replacing them with something better could help them look and feel younger.

> Most people have no idea they have a sensitivity to
> certain foods. They have no idea that simply removing
> a few foods and replacing them with something
> better could help them look and feel younger.

Here are a few relatively common food allergies and sensitivities. I invite you to read about them carefully. Don't just assume none of these apply to you. Remember my friend from chapter 11? He developed a severe dairy allergy late in his life. It took a while to pinpoint this problem because he had been a healthy milk-drinking, butter-spreading, ice cream-loving person for decades and decades. But things change. We change. Keep this in mind as you read on.

Gluten Sensitivity

"Gluten-free" products are trendy right now, and there's a good reason for that. It's been estimated that up to one-third of the US population is reactive to wheat gluten. If you have read books or articles by Daniel Amen or Josh Axe, you are probably aware that they, and others in the medical profession, believe that we would all be better off if we said goodbye to gluten for good.

I am not sounding an alarm or encouraging everyone to jump on the "goodbye, gluten" bandwagon. I know a lot of healthy people, especially some endurance athletes, who swear by their whole-grain breads and cereals.

What's more, I have seen people go gluten-free only to consume mass quantities of corn- and rice-based products and gain weight because they are eating more carbs. They end up exceeding their carbohydrate threshold. This means they have ingested so many carbs that those "carb calories" are quickly being converted and stored as fat.

Insulin Resistance

Insulin resistance (IR) is a progressive problem. It will get worse if not treated with modifications to one's diet. Basically, IR is synonymous with prediabetes, which occurs when a person's muscle, liver, and fat cells don't respond effectively to insulin. This is a challenge that tends to worsen with age, but lifestyle choices make a huge impact one way or the other. All of us should eat healthfully, but especially those of us struggling with any form of IR. I have seen estimates that place as many as half of all Americans in the IR camp. That percentage tends to be higher among those over age 45.

Please visit your doctor or nutritionist if you suspect you might be prediabetic. If you feel like you are on a blood sugar roller coaster, make an appointment right away. Do you find that your energy level fluctuates wildly on any given day? Do you experience strange cravings? Have you been more susceptible to illness lately? See an expert.

I should point out that even those without insulin-related conditions need to focus on their blood sugar balance. Anyone can experience a blood sugar spike when consuming more carbs than are necessary to meet immediate energy needs. Whenever this happens, the extra glucose produced by the body must be transported and stored somewhere.

That's where our insulin enters the game. Insulin converts those extra carbs into either glycogen (an energy source that's stored in our muscles or liver) or fat. And if our glycogen storehouses are full or we are insulin resistant, fat becomes the primary way the excess is warehoused. (By the way, those glycogen storehouses have limited capacity. Fat cells have no such limits. They can keep growing and growing and growing.)

And here is where I need to sound the alarm bell a little more loudly. If we constantly burden our bodies with excess carbs, our cells can become insulin resistant over time. This means that cells that once stored carbs as glycogen now resist that process. Instead, they force the insulin to store glucose as fat.

If you become insulin resistant, you are at high risk for developing type 2 diabetes as well as heart disease. If you are even the least bit worried or suspicious about this health challenge, please see an expert. A sharp doctor will assess your IR level with a few simple measurements, such as your waist circumference, triglyceride level, HDL cholesterol level, blood pressure, and fasting glucose level. Armed with the right information, you can then decide how to modify your diet to see if you can find respite from your problems.

Once you know the foods that trip you up, you can craft a long-term eating plan that meets your specific needs and accommodates your individual preferences. Over time, you will find that making good choices gets easier. After all, finding a leaner, healthier, and more energetic you is great motivation.

21

Readers, Digest!

know many people who have an assortment of digestive problems. In my experience, many of these woes can be fixed—without a trip to the doctor.

If you struggle with digestive issues, here is your first to-do item: Get rid of sodas. Don't drink them. Ever. I know this is a hard line, but even the low- and no-calorie varieties of pop simply are not good for you.

Second, don't wolf down your food. You are not a wolf, after all. Taste it. Chew it. Enjoy it. If you tend to eat as if you were in a time trial, you will be amazed at how much better you feel when you take it slow. You will experience less indigestion and less stress. And you won't "overshoot the runway" in your eating. Many of us in the personal training world use this phrase to describe people who eat so fast, they don't allow their bodies' natural sense of satiety to kick in. And this is a major reason why so many Americans overeat—meal after meal after meal.

> If you tend to eat like you are in a time trial, you will be amazed at how much better you feel when you take it slow.

Third, experiment with some of the various natural digestive aids you might have heard about lately.

I drink mint tea with some fresh ginger zested into it after almost every meal. I also eat plain Greek yogurt with fresh berries mixed in several times a week. These practices have completely overhauled my digestion.

I have friends who swear by kombucha or similar beverages. The key is to explore options and find what is best for you.

Every morning after my calisthenics, I drink some water with honey, lemon, and cinnamon mixed in. Then I eat two forkfuls of fermented sauerkraut. (I can sense you grimacing right now, but try it.) I have been following most of these practices religiously for several months now, and my digestion has improved dramatically.[1]

Further, the probiotics, or "good gut bugs," provided by kombucha, yogurt, and kefir help your body rebalance its proper gut bacteria levels. This helps with not only your digestion but also your nutrient absorption and overall metabolism. This means that your body will be more efficient at burning fat and aiding your efforts to lose weight.

More Than Food and Drink

We put an enormous amount of emphasis on what we put into our bodies through our mouths. And we should. We should pay careful attention to everything we eat and drink. Along with oxygen, these things we consume fuel our billions and billions of regenerating cells. The good news is that whatever we put into our bellies goes through amazing filters, such as the intestines, liver, and kidneys.

However, what about the stuff that gets into our bodies without much filtering? Think about the lotions and other topicals we put on our skin, into our hair, on our lips, and so on. These substances can enter our fatty tissues and, in trace amounts, even our bloodstreams.

I have not seen much conclusive research, but some medical professionals are concerned that common products contain chemicals and preservatives that could be harmful to our bodies. And I am not talking about what a blogger is saying on social media. I am talking about research-based articles in reputable publications.[2]

---

[1] By the way, if you are interested in making your own fermented kraut, see the great recipe in Dawn Stoltzfus and Carol Falb, *From the Farmhouse Kitchen* (Eugene, OR: Harvest House, 2018), 215.

[2] For example, see Markham Heid, "5 Things Wrong with Your Deodorant," *Time*, July 5, 2016, http://time.com/4394051/deodorant-antiperspirant-toxic/.

As I have said many times in this book and continue saying, talk to your doctor. She or he should be up to speed on the latest findings. I am not trying to be an alarmist; I am saying that it is well worth your while to study what you are putting into your body through your skin. Your antiperspirant probably contains aluminum. Your antibacterial soap probably contains triclosan. It's worth talking with a trusted medical professional about these substances and their potential effects on your hormone activity, cancer risk, or reproductive system.

Yes, I caught some grief from my buddies when I shelved my usual deodorant until I found a better choice. But I decided to stop ignoring potentially harmful effects to the only body I will have while I am on planet earth. When in doubt, I go without.

The bottom line is to carefully evaluate what you put into your body. My advice to mind the labels applies to more than just food and drink.

Should You Go "Pro"?

According to a National Health Statistics report, probiotic supplements are the third-most popular nonvitamin supplement sold in the United States.[3]

However, there are many kinds of probiotics in myriad forms—from powders to pills, and from kefir to kombucha with probiotic strains added. So for those of us seeking better digestive help, the question is not just if stomach-friendly bacteria is right for you, but which kind(s) of probiotics. Here are a few guidelines to help you navigate these relatively new waters.

Start Slowly

Like other new health discoveries, probiotics have been hailed as a solution for everything from constipation to allergies to anxiety. However, the early indications are that probiotics' main benefits

[3] Tainya C. Clark et al., "Trends in the Use of Complementary Health Approaches Among Adults: United States, 2002–2012," National Health Statistics Reports, no. 79, February 10, 2015, www.cdc .gov/nchs/data/nhsr/nhsr079.pdf.

are gastrointestinal. I know people with inflammatory bowel disease, abdominal pain and bloating, and diarrhea who have found relief from their symptoms. This makes sense—probiotics interact with our guts' immune cells to help ward off infections and inflammation. It's important to remember that specific types of probiotics work best with specific symptoms. So read package labeling carefully and follow guidelines from your doctor, personal trainer, or other health care professional. For example, in most cases, a supplement should have a CFU (colony-forming unit) count of at least 1 billion but no more than 10 billion to be effective and not cause unpleasant side effects.

Probiotic Versus Antibiotic

Probiotics can be a great idea for us when we are taking an antibiotic. We know that antibiotics kill infection-causing bacteria, but they can also lower the levels of "good bacteria" in our GI tracts. This can create more illness as harmful pathogens flourish in environments that are ill-equipped to fight them. Probiotics can help us keep our bacterial levels balanced and ward off potential problems. However, just as specific probiotics work on specific symptoms, not all probiotics work well with antibiotics. Antibiotics will wipe out some probiotics—right along with those bronchitis germs. If you are prescribed an antibiotic, ask your doctor or pharmacist about the best probiotic solution for your specific circumstances. (Remember that probiotic supplements have a shelf life, just like many other supplements. The longer a product sits on a store's shelves or in your pantry, the more its gut-gracing powers can decrease. So make sure you check the "use by" dates as well as guidelines on how to store various supplements.)

Don't Overdo It

If you are already eating a healthful diet that includes a variety of fermented products (such as yogurt, kefir, kimchi, and kombucha) as well as *prebiotics* like garlic, onions, and leeks, you might not need an additional supplement—or one of the above items with added probiotics mixed in. (A lot of people confuse prebiotics and probiotics. Simply put, prebiotics are what probiotics feed on.)

Additionally, fermented foods and beverages generally contain a greater diversity of microbes than supplements do. This diversity is generally better for your overall health—in part because the fermented foods and beverages provide vitamins, minerals, and other nutrients along with their probiotic benefits.

22

Crush Your Cravings

Has this ever happened to you? It's about 9:00 p.m. You had a pretty good dinner a few hours ago, but you're starting to feel hunger pangs. It's too early to head for bed, and your stomach is rumbling so loudly, you probably couldn't sleep anyway. So you head for the pantry, foraging for cookies.

Or it's three o'clock on a workday afternoon. It's been too long since lunch, and dinner is still hours away. You wander into the break room and find yourself staring longingly at the vending machine as if it holds the answers to life's biggest questions.

Cravings, especially unfortunately timed cravings, can hamstring even some of the most disciplined eaters. However, there are effective and tasty ways to conquer your cravings.

First, start your day off right with a satisfying breakfast. (See chapter 8 for more about this vital meal.) More specifically, strive to make eggs part of your morning meal—poached, boiled, scrambled, in a breakfast burrito, whatever. The protein and healthy fats in eggs help stimulate satiety hormones in our gastrointestinal tracts. These hormones help manage our brains' responses to temptations to snack later.

Other ideas for a filling breakfast include cottage cheese, Greek yogurt with some nuts or seeds mixed in, or almond butter spread on whole-grain or multigrain toast.

Second, be smart about your sweet tooth. For me, being smart is more than just saying no and turning up my nose at a box of donuts in the break room. Instead, I recommend having sweet and healthful alternatives on hand. Strawberries, for example, taste great and contain both soluble and insoluble fiber. This combo helps us feel fuller longer and keeps things moving through our GI tracts. Why is this important? It produces a steadier release of sugar into the bloodstream, producing a longer-lasting boost to our energy levels.

Blackberries, grapefruit, and oranges also provide a winning combination of both kinds of fiber.

Finally, use science to crush cravings. If you are weary, stressed, or simply bummed out on a Monday afternoon, you might be drawn to a bag of potato chips or a sleeve of cookies. To help you resist the urge, load up on foods high in tryptophan, an essential amino acid that helps our bodies produce the mood-balancing hormone serotonin. (Essential amino acids, by the way, are the ones our bodies don't produce. We must get them from the foods we eat.)

> To help you resist junk food cravings, choose snacks
> that are high in tryptophan, which helps our bodies
> produce serotonin: cheese, pumpkin seeds, lentils,
> pineapple, tofu, and salmon jerky.

It's awesome that many foods high in tryptophan are also great snacks: cheese, pumpkin seeds, lentils, pineapple, tofu, and salmon. (I realize that fresh salmon is not exactly snack food, but several companies make salmon jerky or salmon-based energy bars. Trader Joe's and Alaska's Best are two of the best brands I have tasted.)

Here's another suggestion: Try some fresh veggies with hummus dip. Hummus is so high in tryptophan, it's earned the nickname nature's Prozac. I love dipping vegetables in hummus because the chickpeas help my serotonin levels while the fiber in the vegetables helps me feel fuller and less likely to graze on unhealthy snacks.

Part 2

Exercise and Fitness

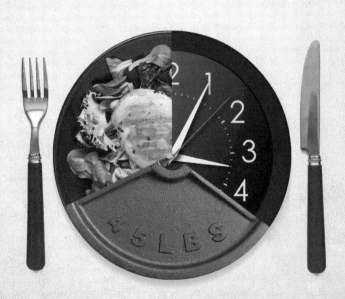

23

Pummel Procrastination

*Procrastination is one of the most common
and deadliest of diseases, and its toll
on success and happiness is heavy.*
WAYNE GRETZKY

Do any of these sound familiar to you?

"Someday I'll start eating better."

"Someday I'll make a doctor's appointment and get a complete physical."

"Someday I'll start exercising regularly again."

"Someday I'll really focus on developing better sleep habits."

Good intentions are fine, but there is a problem with "someday" statements: Sometimes, someday never comes. Opportunities vanish. Disease sets in. People become so out of shape and unhealthy that they reach a point of no return.

Heaven knows life can be busy. But it's your life, and it's up to you how you will spend it. Don't let opportunities to become a healthier person slip through your fingers.

Heaven knows life can be busy. But it's your life, and it's up to
you how you will spend it. Don't let opportunities to become
a healthier you slip through your fingers.

Make an effort. Identify your priorities. Set some time limits if you must. Make that medical appointment. Get rid of that junk food in the pantry. Buy the gift, or if you can, make the gift. Make the effort part of the deal. Put your name on the volunteer list and get committed. Do something kind for the adorable little kid in your life while he or she is still little. Go for a walk together. Teach him or her to play a sport or build a fort. Get some fresh air. Get your hands dirty.

When it comes to exercise, fitness, and other key areas of your life, don't look at time as a prison. Think of it as a gift. Then as you sort through your life's priorities, decide how you want to use this gift of time. Are you going to seize those opportunities to do good (for yourself and others) or neglect them?

> Do all the good you can,
> By all the means you can,
> In all the ways you can,
> In all the places you can,
> At all the times you can,
> To all the people you can,
> As long as ever you can.
>
> OFTEN ATTRIBUTED TO JOHN WESLEY

24

Give Yourself a Good Talking-To

We become the stories we tell ourselves.
ATTRIBUTED TO MICHAEL CUNNINGHAM

The quote above is one of my favorites. Our self-talk is vital to our success in life, but it can also undermine our efforts.

As you strive to become a healthier person, I encourage you to avoid believing lies about yourself, especially lies that come from your own mind. Tell yourself a positive story. In fact, tell yourself many positive stories. As often as you can.

I am here to tell you that positive self-talk works when it comes to exercise, competition, and beyond. It's not a squishy, feel-good fad. A 2014 National Center for Biotechnology Information study revealed that positive self-talk helps athletes perform better and longer and lowers their RPE (rate of perceived exertion). In other words, the athletes who practiced positive self-talk performed better but didn't feel as tired or in as much pain as those in the control group.

In the study, researchers split participants into two groups and asked them to complete cycling time trials to the point of exhaustion. Then for the next two weeks, one group was educated about positive self-talk and instructed to develop motivational statements they could rely on in future time trials. The control group received no such instruction.

When the subjects returned to complete another bike test, the positive self-talk group lasted 18 percent longer than before. The control group's performance didn't improve. What's more, the "self-talkers" ranked their perceived exertion as easier than on their first ride. This is particularly significant because it means the task felt easier even though participants actually biked longer before reaching exhaustion.[1]

It's no surprise that many world-class athletes practice positive self-talk. Ryan Hall is an Olympic marathoner and the US record holder in the half marathon. Hall has several messages he tells himself while competing. One is his version of Proverbs 23:7: "As a man thinks in his heart, so is he."

In various interviews, Hall has shared that this Old Testament wisdom helps him toe the starting line with this assurance: "I have already accomplished my goal for the race."

I encourage you to adopt this practice. Create messages you can give yourself throughout the day, not just during hard workouts. I know people who use various triggers to recite their positive messages. Some do it while brushing their teeth. Others when showering or using the restroom. I know one guy who recites the following Scripture every time he starts his car: "He who began a good work in you will bring it to completion at the day of Jesus Christ" (Philippians 1:6 ESV).

I know a woman who has programmed her smartphone to beep in the middle of the day. This serves as a prompt for her to tell herself, "Today I am focusing on loving God with all my heart. I am loving my family, friends, and coworkers as myself."

Your mind will believe what you tell it most often.

Notice that all these examples are positive. This is so important, especially in this age of negativity and ubiquitous social media critics and trolls. Don't let your self-talk become self-defeating. If I am struggling in the middle of a long run, I don't tell myself, "Don't quit, you

---

[1] A.W. Blanchfield et al., "Talking Yourself Out of Exhaustion: The Effects of Self-Talk on Endurance Performance," National Center for Biotechnology Information, 2014, https://www.ncbi.nlm.nih.gov/pubmed/24121242.

wuss!" No, it's "Power up!" or "C'mon, you're already halfway home. You got this!"

Remember the biblical proverb that Ryan Hall shared. Its truth is undeniable. Your mind will believe what you tell it most often. And your feelings and your behavior will reflect what you believe. So believe the best about yourself. Speak the best about yourself.

25

Outfox Failure

Are you driving your life, or is someone or something else in the driver's seat? This is important to consider when it comes to the topics we're exploring in this book.

We are all imperfect creatures, of course. We all fail sometimes. But I want to help you fail less by answering two key questions: Why do we fail when it comes to our health? And what can we do to avoid failing?

Here's some good news if you have stumbled in your quest to be a healthier person. Every successful person you can think of has failed. Many times. In this book, we talk a lot about how failure and rejection can become the fuel for the drive for success. If you are even a casual basketball fan, you have probably heard that Michael Jordan, perhaps the greatest player ever, played on his high school's junior varsity team as a sophomore. When he was inducted into the Basketball Hall of Fame, he mentioned this disappointment. It still bothered him, but it didn't bring him down. Instead, Jordan channeled his frustration and disappointment into a fierce will to win.

So the big question is not if you will fail, but how you will react to your inevitable failings. What caused you to gain those ten pounds? Why did you go from champ to couch potato? I encourage you to use setbacks like these as learning tools to improve yourself.

When we have a goal, we don't set out to fail. We have the best of intentions. We have a general idea of how to reach our goal. But outside interferences or our own mistakes or doubts hijack our efforts.

Have you ever been typing an email or report for work and placed your hands on the incorrect keys? If so, you know the result. Your intentions were good. You thought you were making the right key-strokes, but one small error messed up everything! This is how I feel when my diet has gone off the rails for a week or when I've skipped one day of exercise, then the next day, and then the next.

During my years as a competitive athlete, coach, and trainer, I have identified a few key traits that can lead to failure. I hope by sharing these, I can help you avoid failure as much as possible—but overcome it when it happens.

Lack of a Clear Goal

Imagine working on your jump shot without a hoop and back-board. How can you know your aim is true? We all need a goal to aim for. I can't count the number of friends, relatives, and personal train-ing clients who have a vague fitness goal, such as "I think I would like to get in better shape and maybe lose a few pounds or something." If you have a kinda-sorta goal, your efforts toward that goal will be half-hearted and unfocused.

> If you have a kinda-sorta goal, your efforts toward that goal will be halfhearted and unfocused.

Lack of Ambition

You need some fire to achieve any important goal, and what goal is more important than caring for your health and well-being? That's foundational to almost everything you do in life. Sometimes you have to really want something to chase it with passion. I urge you to pur-sue better health as if your life depends on it. It does. You have people who love you. You have talents that can make this world a better place. Let that drive you.

Lack of Self-Discipline

If you do not conquer self, you will be conquered *by* self. You need self-control when it comes to your diet, your exercise plan, and your sleep schedule. I can't sugarcoat this: Self-control is a daily battle. Every day you need to fight those negative messages that lurk around you and inside you. Every day you have to overcome your excuses and the legitimate roadblocks life seems to present.

Procrastination

We talked about this in chapter 23, but I have found that procrastination is the number one reason many people fail. So many people say things like "I'm going to start exercising when the New Year arrives" or "I'm going to start eating right as soon as I eat all the junk food in my pantry. Why throw away perfectly good food?"

Procrastination is a wily enemy. "I'll start my exercise program tomorrow" can very easily morph into "I'll start my exercise program next week." You can see where this road leads, right?

Let's face facts. There will never be a "right time" in the future. There will always be a fridge full of excuses. There will always be a couch cushion with your name (and your imprint) on it. Don't wait. Use the resources you have on hand and start moving toward a better future. Now.

Let me give you a real-life example. I had a friend who told me, "I am going to start running as soon as I can get to the store to buy a good pair of running shoes." I looked at the shoes this guy was wearing and told him, "The shoes you have are pretty good. They don't look worn at all. You could start running today. You'll be fine. You can switch to your new shoes as soon as you buy them."

Lack of Persistence

Failure wilts under the heat of good old-fashioned grit. Many of us are good at starting something. We sign up for the two free weeks at the gym. We go out and buy the new running shoes. But then we prove to be lousy finishers. Why? Because we quit at the first sign of resistance.

"The gym was too crowded and noisy when I went. I think I'll come back later."

"Whoa! I went to the Nike store, but I didn't realize athletic shoes had gotten so expensive. I think I'll go home, do some research online, and buy my shoes later when I'm better informed."

I encourage you to avoid nurturing excuses like these. You want to go for a run but it's raining? Wear a hat and watch your step.

By recognizing the roadblocks above, you are more likely to avoid failure. But when you do fail, use failure as a lesson, a kick in the pants to keep moving. Failure, after all, is part of the process. In all fields, people make mistakes every day. Everyone fails at some things sometime.

Recognize those failures but don't let them wrestle you to the ground and choke you. Evaluate what happened. Adapt. Make better decisions. Turn that failure into something better. Give yourself constructive criticism rather than drown in self-loathing. Keep chasing dreams. Keep pursuing goals.

Allow yourself to benefit from trial and error. Stay true to your goals. Value yourself as God's creation, as this will help you when your diet or exercise plans break down. You will triumph. Keep telling yourself that. And keep believing it.

26

Don't Fight a Losing Battle

imagine that soon after the first scale was invented, people began obsessing over how much they weighed. That obsession continues today thanks to digital scales that can give us our weight in pounds and kilograms and include several decimal points.

This might seem like weird advice from a fitness instructor and competitive athlete, but I encourage you to avoid worrying too much about your weight. I often tell people, "Believe the scale less and the mirror more. And believe the way you *feel* even more. Weighing less is way less important than you think."

I am not saying you should completely disregard your body weight. It can be one measure of your progress. I'm simply asking you to stop being obsessed about your weight. If you step on a scale several times a day, you're obsessed. If you know that the scales at your house, your best friend's house, and your gym don't agree with one another, you're obsessed.

Remember those photos I encouraged you to take back in the introduction? Trust those more than your scale. Trust your journal if you keep one. Trust that favorite pair of jeans. And most of all, trust what your body is telling you.

I might seem to be taking a hard stance here, but I have seen way too many people become deeply discouraged by numbers on a scale. Some of them get so discouraged, they give up trying to exercise and eat well. It doesn't have to be that way. It shouldn't be that way.

Here's why. First, muscle weighs more than fat. Muscle makes up more than half of the average person's body weight. I have seen people lose fat while building muscle. But because they don't see those scale numbers plummeting, they conclude they are not making any progress.

Second, our bodies are composed mostly of water—on average, about 55 percent for women and 60 percent for men. This can create myriad traps. On one hand, people go on diets that dehydrate them and think they are dropping fat. They're not. They are just losing water weight. Others will go on a long run (12 miles or so) and report "losing" five or six pounds. I don't disbelieve the totals; after all, some people lose as many as ten pounds during a marathon. But again, it's almost all water.

On the other hand, if you overhydrate or find yourself retaining fluids, you can step on the scale and panic. And if you're a woman, you probably know all about "period pounds," those five pounds or so that can haunt you every month. No wonder so many people think their efforts to eat well and exercise faithfully are not paying off.

One reason for this frustration is that many people misunderstand the difference between weight loss and fat loss. I will explain.

When I step on my bathroom scale, my body weight is the total of my body tissues, what I am wearing, and what is in my stomach, bladder, and intestines. As you know if you've ever fallen into the trap of obsessive weighing, these variables can affect the numbers that pop up on the scale. That's why your weight is probably not the best indicator of your health.

Indeed, the most changeable aspect of your weight is your body water, and that total can rise or fall any day. If you've just worked out hard and sweated buckets, you will weigh less than you did after a large meal, during which you downed four large glasses of water—especially if you haven't had a chance to visit the bathroom yet.

And here is another weighty, water-related matter: The carbs in your body are stored with water. So let's say I go on a hard-core low-carb diet (something I don't often recommend). My carbohydrate reserves will start to drop, as will the water that was stored with those carbs. Initially, I will see an encouraging drop in my body weight. However, this doesn't mean I have lost any fat at all. Losing weight does not equal losing fat.

If you want to accurately track your fat-burning process, you need something that measures your body-fat level. There are several high-tech methods that are accurate but often tedious and expensive, including dual X-ray anthropometry and bioimpedance and underwater weighing.

If you want to go low tech, you can try skin-fold thickness measuring using those dreaded calipers. This method can be somewhat accurate if done correctly, but I don't know anyone who enjoys getting skin pinched on his or her thighs, hips, abs, and so on. In fact, you might be thinking, "You lost me at 'calipers.'"

That's why I favor even more old-fashioned indicators, such as asking myself, "How do my favorite jeans fit?"

Remember that losing a pound of weight doesn't necessarily mean losing a pound of fat. As we have seen, it's relatively easy to lose a pound of water weight, especially if you exercise in the heat. But this loss is temporary, and it doesn't improve your health or fitness. In fact, losing too much water weight can put you at risk of dehydration, which can be dangerous.

> It's relatively easy to lose a pound of water weight, especially if you exercise in the heat. But this loss is temporary, and it doesn't improve your health or fitness.

So be a winner at losing. Be smart. Don't be lured by fad "You can lose a pound a week!" diets. I tell people all the time, "The scale can lie to you—even when it's telling the truth."

If you are eating right and exercising faithfully, take heart. If you are building muscle in places you didn't have much muscle before (especially the legs, buttocks, and back), that new muscle might offset the fat you have shed. And if you are well hydrated (and haven't visited the restroom) when you step on the scale, your results will be skewed even more.

So please stop obsessing about how much weight you have gained or lost, especially in a week or even a month. Keep doing the right things. Keep looking in the mirror. Keep paying attention to how your clothes fit.

Even more important, pay attention to how you are moving, how you are feeling. If the answer to both is "better," you are probably on the right track. And if that special someone in your life starts complimenting you more and asking to feel those new muscles, you are *definitely* on the right track.

Ignore the Myths and Misconceptions

I cringe at the gym when I hear somebody say, "Today I am going to do all my fat-burning exercises."

Sometimes, one of my buddies will demand, "Show me your best fat-burning moves." Then I have to (tactfully) explain the muddled thinking behind this concept.

No wonder so many health myths are flying around these days. Anyone can start a fitness blog and proclaim himself or herself to be an expert.

Plus, there is always a new "revolutionary exercise breakthrough" making the news. The latest discoveries tend to create buzz and get more clicks than solid truths that are backed by years of research.

Other times, the science is basically good, but the results are over-hyped or taken out of context. For example, if a study's subjects are all young world-class athletes, the results might not be applicable to elderly people facing disease or disability.

What's more, exercise physiology is a relatively new field. That's why context is important. No one should change all his or her health habits based on one study. When there is money to be made, there will be people who want to stretch findings and recommendations beyond what is reasonable.

For example, it's no secret that the United States is the fattest nation on earth, and that's why so many people are desperate to lose weight—"Right now, and quickly, please! I am going on a beach vacation next month, and I want to look *hot!*"

Is it any surprise that so many store shelves are crowded with "rapid fat loss" powders, potions, and pills?

I roll my eyes whenever I see an ad for one of those reality shows based on rapid weight loss and muscle gain. This approach is not realistic and not safe for most people. I understand that normal people losing weight and getting in shape at a slow, steady rate does not make for good TV, but it does make for better and longer-lasting results.

This brings us back to those "fat-burning exercises," which is a catch-22 and an oxymoron rolled up in one. I'll explain what I mean. The exercises that burn the most fat, as a percentage of your total available "fuel," are also the exercises that burn the fewest calories per minute.

> The exercises that burn the most fat, as a percentage of your total available "fuel," are also the exercises that burn the fewest calories per minute.

Our bodies use fat for low rates of energy expenditure. That's just the way the human metabolism works. So if you are alive, even your most low-key activities use fat to make energy—even sleeping. But regardless of what some people say, sleeping is *not* the ultimate fat-burning activity. Sleeping burns fat at a sloth-slow rate, and most of us can't spend most of our lives sleeping, as tempting as that might sound on some days.

Because we want results fast, we tend to favor the exercises that burn calories the quickest. And this, as you have probably deduced by now, means we burn a *lower* percentage of fat when compared to other fuel, like glycogen. I wish people didn't worry so much about which fuel they are burning. Our bodies are wonderfully designed. If we don't work against our design, our bodies will replenish fuel according to our built-in priorities.

That's why I am wary of no-carb or ultra-low-carb diets. It's possible for a person on such a diet to get inadequate levels of carbohydrates to replace his or her glycogen level. For most of us, eating a normal diet will keep our glycogen levels where they should be.

Some of this information might seem counterintuitive, but it's simply the way our bodies work.

Here are the most important takeaways from this chapter:

- Don't obsess about fat-burning exercises unless you are an ultra-endurance athlete.
- *Any* exercise that burns calories, builds muscle, and strengthens your heart is good exercise.
- If you are healthy and exercising at a high level, don't carb starve yourself. Eating a reasonable amount of nutrient-dense, complex carbs will help you replace the glycogen you burn.
- Vigorous exercise generally uses more glucose.
- Less vigorous (aerobic) exercise generally burns more fat because there is plenty of oxygen available to help our bodies use fat for energy. This kind of exercise tends to conserve our bodies' supplies of glycogen.

Please keep these points in mind. As I close this chapter, I want to connect what we've covered to my analogy from the introduction about the bow and arrows. Don't let confusion over terms like "fat-burning exercise" or "aerobic versus anaerobic exercise" prevent you from taking aim at better health. Do *something*. Set your goals and start working toward them. You can adjust your aim as you go.

28

A Killer Bod Is Not Worth Dying For

You probably see them everywhere you go—the mall, the pool, the multiplex…just about everywhere but the library. They are the hard-body hotties. The genetic marvels who have been blessed with toned muscles, perfect skin, and digestive systems that apparently burn fat the way a Porsche Turbo Carrera burns fuel.

And when you can't see these physical wonders in person, they still haunt you, smiling at you and flexing for you on TV, magazine covers, websites, and giant billboards. It's intimidating. Sometimes it's downright depressing.

Guys wish, "Why can't I get my abs to pop like that dude's? And look at those arms—they're bigger than my legs!"

Girls wonder, "Could I *ever* starve myself enough to get as thin as that woman? And it should be illegal to have legs that long and toned!"

You may ponder how you can compete with all the buff bods without getting all "jacked" yourself. How can you compete personally or professionally in the sea of bulging biceps, long legs, and perfect pectorals?

Relax. Guys, stop flexing, okay? You don't need to impress anybody right now, and you're gonna get a cramp if you don't chill. Women, no need to keep sucking in your gut; you're among friends now.

Before you buy an expensive piece of exercise equipment from a shop-at-home channel or blow hundreds of dollars on questionable nutritional supplements, you need to consider a few facts.

First, those magazine supermodels and social media stars you envy aren't as perfect as they look. Posters and photos are retouched, airbrushed, filtered, and manipulated in all sorts of ways. Blemishes and wrinkles are removed. (For that matter, *pores* are removed!) Flabby arms are made trim; weenie arms are bulked up. And check this—makeup is used to make guys look like they have washboard abs when in reality, they don't.

And the oils. Let's not forget the oils, which are applied liberally to highlight every sinew, every vein. Sure, you might want to hug these gleaming bods, but they'd probably squirt right out of your arms. (Warning: Don't get any ideas about this oil thing. Don't sneak into the kitchen and try to "Wesson up" your biceps or your legs or your whatever. You're just going to make a mess, stain your clothes, and waste good money. Someone in your house needs that oil for cooking, okay?)

Even the people who look great without all the gimmicks often get their shine on at a high personal cost. For example, steroids pump you up, but they also might alter your personality—and not in a good way. They can make you short-tempered and violent. They can make you sterile or even kill you. And don't think the legal supplements (like some magic "fat incinerators") are necessarily safer. You've probably seen news stories about side effects and trips to urgent care. Just because you can find something on the shelves of your local nutrition store and professional wrestlers endorse it doesn't mean it's safe for you to ingest. Getting a killer bod isn't worth killing yourself, is it?

Granted, having a hottie body might get you noticed at the gym or on your favorite dating site. But if you want an actual relationship, you must have something more to offer than delicious deltoids. After all, gorillas are powerful and physically intimidating, but you don't see them getting lots of dates. (Unless it's with other gorillas.)

Once you've captured someone's attention, you're going to need to *keep* that attention if you want to have a meaningful relationship. You need more than sinew, teeth, and hair. You need a heart that cares, a mind that thinks and wonders, and a soul that reflects heavenly light. When someone asks your boyfriend or girlfriend or spouse, "What is that magic 'something' that sparked the romance between the two of you?" do you really want the answer to be, "Well, more than anything else, it was the 5 percent body fat number!"

Of course, there's nothing wrong with wanting to be fit. Your body is a temple after all, not a Porta-Potty. A balanced diet is a good idea, but a celery stick in each hand is not a balanced meal. The same principle applies to a couple of canned "protein shakes" filled with chemicals most of us can't pronounce.

> Keep your fitness goals in perspective. Don't become obsessed with your body image at the expense of your friendships, your job, your academic career, or your life goals.

A sensible workout program is a good idea too, but do it for the right reasons. Do it to be healthy, not to be a date magnet. If you want to improve your fitness level, check with a doctor—especially about herbal supplements and their pros and cons. (In other words, don't buy your supplements from that hairy guy named Fabiano who wears lots of gold chains and hangs out by the drinking fountain at your local gym.)

Finally, keep your fitness goals in perspective. Don't become obsessed with your body image at the expense of your friendships, your job, your academic career, or your life goals. After all, someday your muscles are going to lose some of their size and tone, no matter how hard you try to prevent it. But if you live well, your relationships, your mind, and your dreams can keep right on growing.

29

Change Your Health by Changing Your Mind

I doubt the apostle Paul was talking about his exercise regimen when he wrote, "For what I am doing, I do not understand; for I am not practicing what I *would* like to do, but I am doing the very thing I hate" (Romans 7:15 NASB). But these words seem apropos when it comes to the way we eat and exercise (or fail to exercise).

A lot of us know what to do to improve our health. The struggle is actually doing it or doing it with any degree of consistency. Our friends or even a trainer or doctor might offer a simple solution: "Just summon your willpower. Come on—motivate yourself."

But it's not that simple. So many people have a love/hate relationship with food, exercise, and even their doctors. Often, we need to get to the core of our issues before we can make lasting changes. And at this core, we might find a tangled knot of unhealthy thinking, bad habits, and self-sabotaging attitudes.

Let's look at a few of these deeper mindsets.

"It's all or nothing."

We touched on this trap earlier. A person can tell himself, "I'm not going to start working on my health until I find the perfect diet, the perfect workout regimen, and the perfect personal trainer or nutritionist." This attitude brings along the pressure of researching the best foods and nutritional supplements, finding the perfect gym, and buying the best shoes and other workout gear. Nothing is wrong with such research, of course, but it shouldn't become an end in itself.

What's more, some people also think they need the perfect time to launch their lifestyle change. They want to wait until they finish a big project at work. Or until after the holidays. Or when the New Year rolls around.

You can see how this attitude can become a roadblock, right? If I think I can't start working on my health until my life is completely organized and I can do everything just perfectly, I'll never get off the starting line.

The truth is that I don't have to be on an official program to make progress. If I decide to get out the door and run a couple of miles today, "just because," my body will benefit just as much as if I ran the same distance with a personal trainer and while wearing my official gym uniform. Every small step in the right direction makes a difference. Those steps don't need to be on your official schedule and sanctioned by your gym or personal trainer.

> If you take three steps forward and two steps back,
> you are still making progress.

Life is messy. We can't always control our food choices or workout options. Sometimes we have to do the best with what we have. Sometimes we will mess up, but we must forgive ourselves and move on. If you take three steps forward and two steps back, you are still making progress. And you are still trying. I encourage everyone I know to focus more on those forward steps than the ones in the wrong direction.

"I always fail. Why bother?"

This mindset is the result of years of failed attempts. After a while, the only exercise someone gets is wallowing in doubt and discouragement.

I know plenty of successful people who encountered failure before finally achieving lasting success. My own story is like this. After enduring physical, financial, and relationship setbacks, I can promise you that the only way you will fail permanently is if you stop trying, stop training, stop learning.

I encourage you to attack every opportunity for even the smallest victory and then celebrate that victory. More important, be thankful for it. Living gratefully is one of the best ways to be a healthy person on every possible level.

You're reading this book right now—that's an accomplishment. That's progress. (By the way, thank you for reading!)

Do what you can each day. Be patient with yourself. Give yourself some grace. Maybe you have failed before. Leave those failures in the past, where they belong. This time can be different.

"It's now or never."

In today's society, we want what we want, and we want it *now.* The next time you're surfing the web or reading a magazine or taking a road trip, note the language of the ads you see. Watch for words like "instant," "quick and easy," and "right now."

Some people seem to believe they can buy exercise in a bottle or take a pill that miraculously burns fat while they watch TV. It's a lie.

A person who is obese didn't get that way overnight. A person who is woefully out of shape didn't lose all that muscle tone, strength, flexibility, and endurance over a holiday weekend. It's a long journey from good health to bad. The same is true of the reverse trip.

The quality of our existence and our ability to live out our life's purpose tomorrow will be affected by the choices and efforts we make today. Our health affects every area of our lives. So it's worth the effort. It's worth the time.

I want to make one more point about the quick-fix attitude. Let's say one of those magic muscle-building, fat-burning pills actually worked. Do we really think this would help people live healthier lives? Or would people binge eat unhealthy foods and binge watch TV all the time, knowing they could rely on that magic pill when they needed it?

Compare this fantasy to health and fitness you earn—something you work for, strive for, and pray for. We value what we earn. I encourage you to keep earning your health and vitality every day. You will be rewarded, and you will build lifestyle habits that will help you be your best, now and in the future. It's never too late to change.

Of course, there are other destructive attitudes, but these are some of the most common. I encourage you to develop a better, healthier attitude. One that says, "My life is a gift from God. So I am going to make the best possible choices, not because I have to, but because I want to. My past failures are just that—past. I have learned from them. Now I am moving forward. Every day is a chance for progress. Some days, that progress will be uneven and messy, but it's still progress. I might not be all I should be yet. But, thank God, I am not who I once was."

30

Rock Your Walk

You may be unlikely to join a gym, hire a personal trainer, or take up a sport. Even though I recommend these things, you can still make yourself healthier without a gym, without fancy equipment, or even without a workout partner. Just get yourself a good pair of walking or running shoes and get out the door!

I recommend 150 minutes of exercise a week. That might sound like a lot, but it's only 25 minutes a day, six days a week. Almost anyone can do that. It's less time than a 30-minute sitcom or local news program.

Walking gobbles calories, increases your circulation, builds muscles, and burns fat. And if you walk outside, you get the added benefits of fresh air and sunshine.

But the benefits don't end there. I have some friends and relatives who see a therapist or psychologist. Some of these mental health professionals prescribe outdoor hiking because it reduces *rumination*— that continuous fixation on troubling or worrisome thoughts. We all know the cycle: The more we focus on bad thoughts, the more we feel anxious and depressed. Then we worry about our depression, and...we know where this road leads.

Walking or hiking, especially out in God's creation, reduces our negative focus. A simple change in location and activity can change our mood. Have you heard the term "ecotherapy"? This is what it's all about.

We've already learned that walking two miles burns about as many calories as running two miles. What's more, a good vigorous walk releases the same endorphins (natural, feel-good chemicals) associated with running.

> Walking two miles burns about as many calories as running two miles and releases the same endorphins associated with running.

I invite you to try rocking your walk. Just take a ten-minute stroll in the most beautiful place you can find right now. You don't have to go far or be out there a long time. You don't need a bunch of special gear. (Although I do encourage you to invest in a good pair of walking or running shoes. Your feet and your back will thank you.)

According to one study of 140,000 people, those who walked even two hours a week were less likely to die a premature death than their nonwalking counterparts. Further, those who walked more than two hours weekly had even better health than the minimum group.[1]

What's more, for years walking has been shown to reduce the risk of heart disease, diabetes, and certain forms of cancer.

So I encourage you—walk on.

Who's Hungrier, the Fit or Those Who Sit?

If you avoid exercise because you think it will make you hungrier—and therefore more likely to eat more and gain weight—you are about to lose an excuse. In a study at the University of Massachusetts at Amherst, researcher Barry Braun observed the same group of fit young subjects in three one-day experiments.[2]

On the "active day" of the study, the subjects spent 12 hours being physically active—walking, doing laundry, and handling office work such as

---

[1] Alpa Patel et al., "Walking in Relation to Mortality in a Large Prospective Cohort of Older US Adults," *American Journal of Preventive Medicine* 54, no. 1 (January 2018): 10-19; cited in Ana Sandoiu, "Under 2 Hours of Walking per Week May Considerably Prolong Life," *Medical News Today*, October 19, 2017, https://www.medicalnewstoday.com/articles/319785.php.

[2] Cited in Rob Stein, "The Checkup," *Washington Post*, September 30, 2008, http://www.washingtonpost.com/wp-dyn/content/article/2008/09/26/AR2008092603105.html?noredirect=on.

sorting documents and picking up books. They were not allowed to sit for more than ten minutes in an hour.

On the other two days, the subjects watched videos and worked only on computers. They could move around only by being pushed in wheelchairs.

They were served the same amount of food on two of the three days, but on the second "sedentary day," the food intake was reduced.

At the study's conclusion, the subjects reported feeling hungrier, having a greater desire to eat, and sensing they could eat more after a meal on the sedentary, couch-potato days than after the highly active day.

31

Don't Put Yourself on the Spot

Almost all of us have places on our bodies where we would like to see less fat. The people who concoct diets, exercise regimens, and revolutionary herbal supplements know this. That's why we see so many ads boasting ways to target our belly fat, or derriere fat, or whatever.

I'm here to report a somewhat depressing fact. There is simply no way to control where fat is lost. We cannot tell fat cells in our thighs, for example, "Okay, this next set of leg presses is coming for you. Prepare to die."

Here are a few basic physiological factors to consider. First, the number of fat cells in our adult bodies is relatively stable. When we put on weight, it's not that we are generating brand-new fat cells. Instead, the problem is that our existing fat cells swell. When we lose weight, the opposite happens.

And here is more sad but true news for hopeful spot reducers. When we diet and exercise, fat loss probably tends to happen first in the cells that are the most recently swollen. In other words, it's probably going to take a while to reduce fat in areas that have been trouble spots for a long time. (I'm talking about you, pot belly. And you too, love handles.)

Do you know people who have gone on a fitness kick and made huge progress in some areas of their bodies, but that "middle-age man gut" hung on for dear life? Or that backside never seemed to back off?

I remember a hefty friend telling me, "I'm going to do hundreds of sit-ups every single day until I get rid of this gut and I have a six-pack. Don't you think that will work?"

I said, "It will work—if your goal is to be a fat guy who can do a lot of sit-ups."

Sadly, there is no scientific or logical reason to think leg exercises will reduce the fat on your legs. Or that targeting your glutes will remove fat from your butt.

Now, exercising a muscle might make it bigger and more toned. But making a muscle bigger and stronger does not have much of an effect on the fat cells in the immediate vicinity. Yes, a larger, more toned muscle might be more visible, but don't confuse muscle growth with fat loss. I know people who have added muscle to their frames but also gained fat because they didn't eat wisely. (Some of them used exercise to justify eating more.)

> Don't confuse muscle growth with fat loss. I know people who have added muscle to their frames but also gained fat because they didn't eat wisely.

I must repeat here what I have said throughout the book: Our goal should be to put ourselves in caloric deficit. We must burn more calories than we ingest. This is what reduces subcutaneous fat (the fat that is just below the skin) and gives us the toned appearance we strive for.

This brings me to the subject of cellulite. Have you seen supplements or exercises touted to blast away cellulite cells? There is only one problem with pitches like this. There is no such thing as a cellulite cell. Really. Cellulite is just the name given to fat cells that have "melded" or integrated with connective tissue. This combination of subcutaneous tissue gives one's skin a bumpy or dimpled appearance.

To the best of my knowledge, cellulite is something of a mystery, even to those of us in health and fitness professions. Some people think cellulite is related to sex hormones because it's way more common in women than it is in men.

There is no true cure for cellulite, and there is certainly no quick fix, despite the boasts of TV and online ads. Don't be shamed by ads like these. Cellulite is not a disease or disorder; it's just not a look people like.

And please don't let this little "reality check" dissuade you from working out. I have good news for you: As you become more fit and reduce the amount of subcutaneous fat in your body, your skin will probably smooth out, and its appearance will change for the better.

As I close this chapter, I want to talk briefly about love handles. As we have learned, you cannot laser target your love handles. However, you can include your love handles among all other trouble spots in your smart, sustainable, and systematic exercise and dietary efforts.

In other words, I encourage you to look at burning fat and building muscle as a way of life. Forget the gimmicks. Forget the crash programs. They don't work. The only thing you'll lose a lot of is your money.

Instead, be steady. Make progress every chance you get. That way, you will look better and feel better all over.

A Good News Gut Check

Whenever I talk to people about the myths of spot reducing, I see a lot of crestfallen faces. And I hear comments like, "You mean I can't lose my beer gut by doing hundreds of sit-ups? That's so depressing!"

Reality checks are not fun to hear. They aren't that fun to deliver either. So I think it's worthwhile to offer a bit of good news on the "tummy troubles" front.

In part 1, I devoted a lot of ink to the value of probiotics for improving your digestive health. As it turns out, improving the metabolic activity in your digestive system can help tighten your core and give you a sexier stomach in the process.

As we have learned, your gut is teeming with trillions of microscopic bacteria. Some of these bacteria are probiotics, part of your immune-defense army. Other bacteria are disease-promoting pathogens (germs!) that create havoc and illness. Think of your probiotics as "friendly bugs," a peacekeeping force striving to maintain your optimal microbial balance. If you don't have enough of these good guys, your immune system and health level may suffer.

Probiotics have allies called prebiotics, which are found in foods like garlic, nuts, wheat, onions, and Jerusalem artichokes. Prebiotics are fuel for probiotics. They fortify your army of beneficial bugs and keep your immune system strong. Right now, there is a battle waging in your gut, and you want the good bacteria to outnumber the enemy so that victory is ensured.

Unfortunately, some foods and beverages contain fermentable carbohydrates that make things worse, not better. For some people, dairy products, high-fructose corn syrup, artificial sweeteners (like sorbitol, xylitol, and mannitol), beans, and even some fruits and vegetables cause (or exacerbate) heartburn, irritable-bowel syndrome, colitis, gas, bloating, and diarrhea. (Incidentally, some brands of protein bars and energy bars are loaded with sugar substitutes. One more reason to "mind the labels.") So identifying possible trouble foods and beverages can reduce or eliminate gas and bloating, which make our midsections appear larger than they really are.

Believe it or not, there's even more good news to digest here. Improving the digestive landscape in your gut can, in some cases, result in a trimmer torso. Here's how friendly gut organisms help fend off fat accumulation around your waistline: When indigestible fiber is fermented in your large intestine, the process releases energy as well as short-chain fatty acids (SCFAs). Your healthy microorganisms enhance the release of energy and the resulting boost to your metabolism. This means your food is used for fuel more efficiently. And as we have learned, food that is burned as fuel doesn't end up as fat along your waistline or anywhere else.

There is research to support this good news. For example, a 2010 study from the *European Journal of Clinical Nutrition* examined the effects of a fermented milk formula on the excess abdominal fat levels (and weight) of 87 overweight subjects. For 12 weeks, the subjects drank about a cup of milk daily, but half of the group had a probiotic strain called *Lactobacillus gasseri* added. At the end of the study, this "probiotic group" enjoyed a 4.6 percent decrease in their abdominal fat, a 1.8 percent decrease in waist circumference, and a 1.4 percent drop in weight. The control group, conversely, saw little to no improvement in any area.[1]

Just one more good reason to "go pro(biotic)" and to keep doing exercises to strengthen and tone your abdominal muscles!

[1] Y. Kadooka et al., "Regulation of Abdominal Adiposity by Probiotics (Lactobacillus gasseri SBT2055) in Adults with Obese Tendencies in a Randomized Controlled Trial," National Center for Biotechnology Information, March 10, 2010, https://www.ncbi.nlm.nih.gov/pubmed/20216555.

32

Exercise and Eat Smarter

Have you ever eaten a rich dessert and thought, "Well, I have just made myself fatter" or "That donut is going right to my backside."

Most of us have thoughts and worries like these: "How will the foods I eat affect how I look?" But we don't spend enough time thinking about how the foods we eat affect how we think—how our brains function. Many of us worry about Alzheimer's disease or other forms of dementia but make no connection to diet or exercise.

Right now, there is no guaranteed safeguard against Alzheimer's disease. However, there is much you can do to keep your brain sharp without spending a lot of money.

Research on keeping one's brain sharp is encouraging, although preliminary. However, here are a few of the things we are learning. Getting physical exercise and stimulating your mind with various brain games and activities seem to keep one's brain nimble and functioning at higher levels.

> Getting physical exercise and stimulating your mind with various brain games and activities seem to keep one's brain nimble and functioning at higher levels.

For example, Dr. Kenneth Langa, a dementia expert at the University of Michigan, notes, "I've been recommending these kinds of things [exercise, reading, and brain games and activities] to my patients for several years."[1]

---

[1] Cited in Linda Johnson, "Trying to Keep Brain Sharp Doesn't Have to Be Costly," *Washington Times*, July 12, 2017, https://m.washingtontimes.com/news/2017/jul/12/trying-to-keep-brain-sharp-doesnt -have-to-be-costl/.

Langa is one of the leaders of a National Institute of Aging study, which has been following the health of 20,000 Americans aged 51 and up for the past 27 years. The study has learned that the rate of newly diagnosed dementia cases has dropped by more than 25 percent during the study. Langa credits much of this progress to the patients' continuing to educate themselves and taking active steps to produce more connections among their brain cells. "People should walk, talk, and read," he says.

More than 5 million Americans struggle with Alzheimer's, which is the most common form of dementia. According to Langa, the lifetime risk is about 15 percent. The next time you are in a group of about 100, look around. About 15 members of that group will face Alzheimer's during their lifetimes.

That news might be depressing, but the good news is that there is much we can do to keep our brains healthy. And the worst thing you can do is to sit on the couch all day, eat junk food, and watch junk TV.

Conversely, mental stimulation reduces the rate of mild cognitive impairment. Mental stimulation can come in many forms. I highly recommend activity books like Mary Eakin's *Mind Delights* and *Brain Snacks* (Harvest House).

Composing an email or researching a topic on the web also stimulates the brain. This is so important because, according to a Mayo Clinic study of aging, people with even mild cognitive impairment are ten times more likely to develop Alzheimer's than others.[2]

That Mayo study tracked the progress of about 2,000 subjects, ages 70 and older, for four years. The subjects who participated in mentally stimulating activities once or twice a week cut their risk of developing mild cognitive impairment by 30 percent.

And here is some more good news for you: It's likely that one of

---

[2] Kenneth Langa et al., "A Comparison of the Prevalence of Dementia in the United States in 2000 and 2012," JAMA Network, January 2017, https://jamanetwork.com/journals/jamainternalmedicine/fullarticle/2587084.

your favorite hobbies or activities will help keep your brain sharp. Here are just a few activities that help.

sewing

knitting (or any form of the "fiber arts")

pottery

attending a play or lecture

playing cards

playing board games

playing electronic word games

doing crossword puzzles, Sudoku, word searches, mazes, and so on

reading books

writing blogs, emails, or cards and letters

Don't Forget to Exercise Your Brain

Most of us know that our muscles need exercise to keep them toned and strong, but the brain often gets shorted in the deal. Your brain needs exercise and stimulation to keep it healthy too. And exercising your brain becomes more important as you age. Here are five exercises to build and maintain your brainpower.

1. *Do the unpredictable.* Routines can become brain ruts. Your brain adjusts to your daily routine and doesn't get as stimulated as it used to. Offset this effect by mixing things up. Change your morning ritual. Take a different route to work or school. If you eat breakfast before you shower and do your morning grooming, change the order.

2. *Declare an occasional Opposite Day.* Brush your teeth with your opposite hand. Use your "off hand" to manipulate your computer mouse, apply aftershave or makeup, or punch in phone numbers.

3. *Learn a new word a day.* Flip through a dictionary or thesaurus to

build your vocabulary, or have your new word emailed to you from www.merriam-webster.com.

4. *Learn a new language.* It's not as hard as you might think, and it could open new worlds for you—and be a boost to your career too. Check out what's available at your local community college, use a system like Pimsler or Rosetta Stone, or investigate online sources, such as www.studyspanish.com.

5. *Give your brain a workout.* Sudoku and crossword puzzles provide a stimulating fitness session for your mind. If you want more variety, check out www.prevention.com/braingames for other ways to strengthen your cerebellum.

33

Exercise Your Right to Be Joyful

Sing a new song to the Lord,
for he has done wonderful deeds.
PSALM 98:1 NLT

Do you remember running through a field at top speed when you were a kid just because you could? Just for the pure joy of going fast? What adventure! To leap, climb, twirl in circles, run, bike at warp speed, and propel oneself through water…these are activities of pure happiness.

Challenging our muscles and cardiovascular system with exercise feels good. How sad that this simple truth has been all but forgotten. In fact, exercise has gotten a bad rap in certain circles.

The truth is that a good workout builds strength, agility, flexibility, and self-confidence. It controls your weight. It helps fight depression and increases your resistance to disease. And you don't have to be a great athlete to enjoy the rush of the 100 percent natural stimulants called endorphins, which are released during aerobic exercise. Yes, being a couch potato can become a habit, but so can the positive, enriching, and ennobling sense of well-being that a rousing game of tennis, a bike ride, or a simple brisk walk provides.

"The body wants to be healthy. This is the natural condition…
When the body is out of balance, it wants to get back to it."
—Andrew Weil

Many seniors are hooked on various medications, but at 82, one man I know is (healthily) hooked on exercise. If Ben finds himself getting a bit grumpy, he knows it's time to take a swim. Afterward, he exudes happiness, proclaiming how much better he feels—thanks to the two miles he swam. He says he feels like he leaves his stress in the depths of the swimming pool. And Ben's commitment to exercise doesn't benefit him alone. He inspires his children and grandchildren, who are shaping up to be lifelong exercise enthusiasts, just like the 82-year-old patriarch.

So be like Ben. Increase your energy levels, invigorate your body, and promote a positive attitude. To exercise is to exhilarate and to encourage feelings of immediate contentment and deep, lasting happiness.

Let's recapture that childhood joy. Let's run, spin, jump, bike, or at least walk for the pure joy that spreads from our well-toned limbs to our minds and souls—which hunger to be refreshed. Let's exercise our right to be healthy…and happy.

Matt's Morning Movements

I enjoy many opportunities to exercise the right to be joyful and healthy, including my "morning movements" routine. I do these movements every morning if possible. These few, simple moves have absolutely changed my life, and I believe they can change yours too. The goal is to drain your lymph nodes and get blood flowing to all your organs and extremities.

What's more, I have found that this routine has made my muscles feel more relaxed and my mind more refreshed. After I have used the bathroom and consumed my morning water/detox concoction, this is my drill. I hope it will become yours as well.

1. Stand tall with your feet shoulder-width apart. Raise your arms above your head as if you are making a snow angel. Stretch your hands toward the ceiling while standing as tall as you can. Next, flex your gluteal muscles hard for about ten seconds as you rise up on your toes. Now gently come down onto your heels. Move your feet closer together and lower your arms, exhaling fully. Repeat this

process five times, focusing on inhaling deeply as your arms come up and exhaling fully as they come back down.

2. Stand with your feet together, your toes spread, and your quads flexed. Your tailbone should point straight down, your shoulder blades should be open fully, and your head should be held high, as if you are standing at attention. While in this posture, breathe deeply and fully, in and out. Breathe from your stomach. Repeat three to five times—or more if you like how it feels.

3. Bonus move. Do some wall slides and scapular push-ups. (Check out Eric Cressey's YouTube videos for great instruction on these moves and many, many others.)

I have found that taking the time to do this quick morning routine has improved my posture and my breathing. And I have less pain in my shoulders and in my hands. I hope you will get in this habit too. If you need to sip a little coffee to help you get going, go right ahead. Just remember to keep breathing deeply, and don't force any movement if it causes sharp pain. Don't beat yourself up if you miss a morning or two. Just get back into the routine as you are able.

34

Give Running a Try (or Another Try)

This is one of two chapters in which I will encourage you to try a form of exercise that many people write off as too old-school or too strenuous, especially for people over 40. I will address weight lifting in the next chapter. This chapter focuses on the many benefits of one of the oldest forms of exercise known to humanity—running.

I have heard people argue, "Running is bad for your knees and bad for your back."

You know what is *really* bad for your joints? Inactivity. Lack of movement. And the obesity that accompanies both.

I urge you to give this simple, inexpensive activity a try (or another try). Running might not be as hard on your joints as you might imagine.

Further, running is wonderful for your circulation and your heart health. Running improves the elasticity and dilation of your arteries. It restores your blood vessels and helps them function at peak levels. Why? Because running causes so many of your muscles to demand oxygen-rich blood—your quads, calves, glutes, lats, shoulders, and biceps, just to name a few.

Picture this: As you run, that oxygen-rich blood flows through your arteries and into your muscle fibers. In the process, you are keeping your arteries strong and healthy. Pumping that blood strengthens your heart too. On the days when it's hard to get motivated or your run isn't going well, focus on all the good things happening inside your body. This always helps me persevere through a difficult workout.

Running's benefits for the arteries and the heart should be great news for those in their AARP years.

In a feature in *Runner's World* magazine, Douglas Seals, a professor of integrative physiology at the University of Colorado, noted, "We now know that cognitive decline with aging and disease are significantly due to decline in artery function and health. Your tendency to become more prone to diabetes with aging is affected and highly correlated with vascular health and function. Even kidney disease is closely linked to the health of your arteries."[1]

As we learned in chapter 32, Alzheimer's and other forms of dementia are a huge concern these days. Great strides are being made in the world of medication and gene therapy, but we have a wonderful tool right now, as the information from professor Seals indicates.

The good news doesn't stop there. Running also challenges your brain. Now, you might think it's a rather mindless activity. Just keep alternating feet, and you are good to go. But running is like tennis or skiing in the way it engages fine motor skills.

On today's run, for example, I had to leap over a bag of garbage someone left on the sidewalk. I had to zigzag to dodge the neighbor's dog, who strained at his leash to greet me. Later, I had to increase my speed to get across an intersection before the light changed.

Running provides challenges for you to navigate. And even if you favor running on a treadmill, you can mix things up by adjusting your speed and incline level—or changing your stride length from time to time.

Running just two hours per week can slash your risk of cardio death by 45 to 70 percent—and your chance of dying of cancer by 30 to 50 percent.[2]

You really don't have to run very long or very far to reap many, many benefits. As a trainer, I have seen people enjoy huge gains in their fitness level, aerobic health, and general appearance with very modest

[1] Cited in Wes Judd, "To Look and Feel Younger, Running Is the Real Miracle Drug," *Runner's World*, February 9, 2018, https://www.runnersworld.com/news/a20865704/to-look-and-feel-younger-running-is-the-real-miracle-drug/.

[2] Judd, "To Look and Feel Younger, Running Is the Real Miracle Drug."

mileage. I am talking about just two to two and a half hours per week. That's only about 20 minutes a day.

That's not a lot of mileage—and not a lot of time investment either. If you run on a treadmill, you could have time to warm up, do your run, and cool down—all within the framework of your favorite half-hour sitcom or sports-talk show.

And here is more good news if you are of a certain age. When it comes to heart health, brain benefits, and disease prevention, you will benefit no matter what your age—40 or 50 or 80.

However, those of us between the ages of 40 and 60 often see the most benefits of a smart running regimen. That's important because this age range is when many of the various age-related diseases and conditions emerge.

I won't get too technical, but running benefits you on a cellular level. More research will need to be done, but it appears that running restores and rejuvenates your mitochondria. From middle school biology, you might recall that mitochondria are the powerhouses of your cells. They give muscle fibers their energy, allowing them to contract and perform efficiently.

> Running appears to stimulate the repair of mitochondria.
> They generate energy efficiently, as they did
> when you were younger.

As we age, our mitochondria become less effective at generating their chemical energy. Running appears to stimulate the repair of mitochondria. They generate energy efficiently, as they did when you were younger. A 2014 University of Colorado study found that older runners had better mitochondrial health than their nonrunning counterparts. And they were more efficient runners as well. This means that they were less likely to be injured and that they were learning to run with less wasted energy.[3]

---

[3] Justus Ortega et al., "Running for Exercise Mitigates Age-Related Deterioration of Walking Economy," *PLOS One*, November 20, 2014, http://journals.plos.org/plosone/article?id=10.1371/journal .pone.0113471.

Here is the bottom line: Running trains your muscles to perform as they did when you were younger. And those healthy mitochondria help you be more active in all aspects of your life. They help you fend off heart disease, diabetes, obesity, bone loss, and more. Wouldn't you love to have the strength, vigor, and energy to do more?

"But what about running and my knees?" you might ask. "What about the joint pain and arthritis sometimes associated with running?"

Recent research is indicating that a moderate amount of running *lowers* inflammation in knee joints. In a study reported in *Time* magazine, subjects had fewer "pro-inflammatory markers" in their knee fluid after a 30-minute run.[4] More evidence for one of this book's mantras: Motion is lotion.

Perhaps you simply can't run for one reason or another. That's okay. But please find an aerobic activity that works for you. Something. Anything. Here is why it is important to find an aerobic activity: Your heart doesn't really distinguish between a bike ride or rowing session that gets your pulse rate up to 120 beats per minute and a run that does the exact same thing.

I hope you are inspired to try running—or retry running.

It's interesting to me that the health and fitness industry keeps producing "magic elixirs" and new, state-of-the-art machines and programs. However, a simple, basic exercise often provides the most and *longest-running* benefits.

[4] Alexandra Sifferlin, "3 Things You Didn't Know About Running," *Time*, June 30, 2017, http://time.com/4825495/is-running-good-for-you/.

35

Weight a Minute

have been lifting weights since I was 11 years old. Guess what? I am in my early forties now, and it didn't stunt my growth (I'm six feet three inches). It didn't damage my bones either.

The mere thought of pumping iron can be intimidating to many people, but I encourage you to rethink weight lifting. For example, when I say weight lifting, I don't limit the term to pumping iron—dumbbells, barbells, and kettlebells. I am referring to body-weight exercises *and* those done with resistance bands and exercise machines. There are many ways to increase strength, burn fat, and build flexibility and balance through resistance training.

I strength train three times a week. Usually, I warm up and then complete two sets of body-pressing exercises followed by two body-pulling exercises. Then I do a few exercises that target my legs and hips.

A typical workout for me includes the exercises below. (Don't worry if you have never heard of some of these. I am including them to show the variety of strength-training moves available.)

glute bridges	one-armed rows
hip thrusts	fat man rows
one-legged deadlifts	chin-ups (using gymnastics rings)
walking lunges	box jumps with a step down
wall handstands (on my fists)	dumbbell curls
kettlebell overhead presses	dumbbell triceps extensions
floor presses with dumbbell	resistance band pull-aparts

shoulder dislocates (for mobility)	kettlebell swings
windmill press	snatches
push-ups	clean and push presses
lateral raises	Turkish get-ups and renegade rows
rear deltoid raises	

On the days in between my strength training, I walk for an hour or so or do a sport. As we'll see in chapter 38, that doesn't mean you have to join some kind of official league. I am really into Brazilian jiujitsu right now, but on many of my "sport days," I play a round of golf or simply hit balls at the driving range for a while. Or I find a batting cage and swat baseballs for a half hour or so. Other times, I swim.

Because I travel a lot and sometimes work in a foreign country, my exercise environment is never perfect. I often find myself in a hotel with lousy exercise equipment, an uncomfortable bed, and terrible food. But I don't let these things stop me. Hard work trumps perfection. I do the best I can with what is available. I use good form even if I'm using bad equipment.

> I often find myself in a hotel with lousy exercise equipment, an uncomfortable bed, and terrible food. But I don't let these things stop me. Hard work trumps perfection.

As I have noted, this is not a scientific textbook on health. However, I do want to briefly explore some of the solid research behind weight/resistance training and dispel some of the myths associated with pumping iron.

First, you don't have to lift heavy weights. You can greatly enhance your physical function and general fitness with some light dumbbells or just your own body weight. As I have noted, the hotels I stay in often have poor equipment or no equipment at all. But I don't stress about this. Doing some push-ups, sit-ups, lunges, squats, and planks in my hotel room works just fine. The important thing is to do *something*.

"To me, resistance training is the most important form of training for overall health and wellness," says Brad Schoenfeld, a professor of exercise science at New York City's Lehman College and also a champion drug-free body builder. Schoenfeld has published more than 30 academic papers on various aspects of resistance training.

Schoenfeld adds, "Bone resorption…is a decrease in bone tissue over time. When you're young, bone resorption is balanced and in some cases exceeded by new bone tissue generation. But later in life, bone tissue losses accelerate and outpace the creation of new bone."[1]

Schoenfeld notes that this acceleration is especially pronounced in people who are sedentary and in women who have reached or passed menopause. This loss of bone tissue leads to the weakness and postural problems that plague many older adults.

Fortunately, resistance training combats these problems. Strength training stimulates the development of osteoblasts, which are cells that rebuild our bone tissue.

I am a big fan of aerobic training, but my years of experience have shown me that resistance training is the best way to maintain and enhance your total-body bone strength. I simply cannot recommend it enough.

What's more, early indications are that resistance training improves insulin sensitivity among people with diabetes and prediabetes. Specifically, twice-weekly training sessions helped control insulin swings and body weight fluctuations.[2] This research mirrors what I have learned and experienced over many years of training. Our muscles are very metabolically active. They use glucose (also known as blood sugar) for energy. When we resistance train, our muscles gobble up glucose. And this glucose consumption continues even after we have finished

[1] Cited in Markham Heid, "Why Weight Training Is Ridiculously Good for You," *Time*, June 6, 2017, http://time.com/4803697/bodybuilding-strength-training/.

[2] N.D. Eves and P.C. Plotnikoff, "Resistance Training and Type 2 Diabetes: Considerations for Implementation at the Population Level," *Diabetes Care* 29, no. 8 (August 2006): 1933–41, http://care.diabetesjournals.org/content/29/8/1933.

exercising. Have you heard the term "afterburn" in relation to exercising? This is one example of the long-lasting effects of physical training.

This is why anyone at risk for metabolic conditions such as type-2 diabetes, high blood pressure, and high cholesterol should investigate the benefits of strength training.

Here's one more reason to try this form of exercise. Strength training might help ward off inflammation, which is a major risk factor for heart disease and many other conditions.[3] A Mayo Clinic study, for example, found that when overweight women did twice-weekly resistance training sessions, they experienced significant drops in several markers for inflammation.[4] Another study at the University of Connecticut showed similar results.[5]

And I want to emphasize one more time that you don't need to lift heavy loads to build muscle, increase flexibility, and strengthen your bones. I have seen people make huge gains with light-load training. Lifting even small weights can have big benefits.

If you're not sure where to begin with your training, I recommend you start with exercises for your back, chest, upper legs, upper arms (biceps and triceps), and abdominal muscles. It's important to think about balance and core strength and stability when doing resistance work. For example, don't focus all your effort on your biceps and your chest, guys. We all need to work the muscles we can't see as well as the usual suspects. Taking an eclectic approach to your workouts will keep your strength in balance, improve your posture, and reduce the risk of injury.

Fair warning: If you haven't lifted weights in a while, the muscles you work are going to be a bit sore. You won't have to guess which

[3] See Mariana C. Calle and Paria Luz Fernandez, "Effects of Resistance Training on the Inflammatory Response," Synapse, August 31, 2010, https://synapse.koreamed.org/DOIx.php?id=10.4162/nrp.2010.4.4.259&vmode=FULL.

[4] Mayo Clinic, "Strength training: Get stronger, leaner, healthier," April 22, 2016, www.mayoclinic.org/healthy-lifestyle/fitness/in-depth/strength-training/art-20046670.

[5] M.C. Calle and M.L. Fernandez, "Effects of resistance training on the inflammatory response," Nutrition Research and Practice 4, no. 4 (2010): 259-69.

muscles you have worked; they will let you know. Of course, if your pain is severe and/or doesn't fade as the days go by, check with a doctor to make sure you haven't injured yourself. This caveat aside, a little soreness is a good thing. It's an indicator that you have done some good work. You have accomplished something.

As you continue to lift, you can minimize soreness by starting your workouts easy and building up gradually. This will also help you get better long-term results by minimizing your risk of injury.

Conquer Injuries

I have been injured a lot. When I was a kid, I was our neighborhood Evel Knievel. We used to build huge ramps and jump our bikes off them. I recall having to visit local garage sales to find new bike frames because I broke a lot of bikes.

One day I decided to jump my bike off the loading dock of our local Kmart. At the last second, I realized I wasn't going fast enough, so I slammed on my brakes to abort my jump. Too late. I toppled over the dock and landed on my head. I can still feel the pain. To my knowledge, that accident didn't have any permanent effects, but it was probably the first of many concussions.

Later, during my senior year of football, disaster struck again. I had been on the field for almost every play—offense, defense, and special teams. My coaches decided to give me a break and take me off the punt team, where I served as the punter. However, after my replacement averaged about three yards a kick in our first two games, I resumed my punting duties.

One day during practice, I stood in the backfield, waiting for the center to long-snap the ball to me. I fielded the snap and prepared to kick the ball. One defender, who happened to be the punter I replaced, dove in front of me. He blocked the kick, but he also crashed onto my leg. My right shin connected with his helmet. I heard the snap of both bones in my lower right leg—my tibia and my fibula.

My leg eventually healed, but it's now more than a half inch shorter than my left leg. As a result, I have had many problems with my left knee and hip. And because the injury affected my circulation, I have experienced blood-flow problems in my right leg and foot.

Injuries have been my constant companion ever since. I dislocated both shoulders many times during my football career. I severed a ligament in my left hand while training for a strongman contest. A major car accident about 18 years ago resulted in back and neck pain that still haunt me today.

I sympathize with anyone who strives to exercise while dealing with injuries or chronic conditions. However, none of us should use injuries as an excuse. We must learn to work around those injuries. We should explore how exercise might actually help.

> None of us should use injuries as an excuse. We must learn to work around those injuries. We should explore how exercise might actually help.

I recently met someone who told me, "I can't even walk for exercise because I have a bad knee." I reminded him, "Motion is lotion. Start walking, just a little bit a day. Try not to sit for more than 45 minutes at a time. Just try to move more and see if your knee—and your back, neck, hips, and shoulders—don't start to feel better."

Another way to treat joint injuries and pain is with a foam roller. These great tools come in a variety of sizes, and they are relatively inexpensive. I use them all the time for my back, quads, glutes, IT band, and more. YouTube has many videos on how to use these tools. You can also use a racquetball or tennis ball to treat foot pain and tightness. My distance-running friends roll a racquetball under their feet to treat and prevent plantar fasciitis.

Of course, you should work with a doctor and/or a physical therapist when you deal with a significant injury, whether it's a new problem or something that has been nagging you for years. The best way to deal effectively with an injury is to pinpoint what it is, and we often need a medical professional for this task.

You might be interested to know that I have been sitting in a hotel room writing this chapter. I began to feel soreness and stiffness in my back and my legs, so I got up and did 40 hip thrusts, using my chair to balance myself. Then I walked up and down the hotel stairs a few times.

The result: I got my glutes firing, and I stretched out my psoas and hip flexors. That always helps with knee pain and stiffness as well as my sore back. What's more, I burned some calories and stoked my internal furnace. I didn't consider this an official workout, just a way to loosen up and clear my head for more writing. And that's a good thing, because I am eager for the next chapter.

Fire and Ice

As we have seen, sometimes our efforts to be healthy can be a strain, especially when we overdo things at the gym, on the volleyball court, or wherever. When you have an aching muscle (or five), you face the age-old treatment dilemma—ice or heat?

The answer depends on what is causing your pain. Generally we use heat to draw blood to a muscle so it will relax and heal more effectively. Heat often works well for chronic minor injuries or conditions, such as a stiff back.

Ice is great for painful muscle inflammation, as it reduces swelling and soreness. Ice is often the preferred treatment for an acute injury suffered within the past 48 hours or so.

When I am talking about heat, I am talking about therapeutic warmth. Extreme heat can burn your skin and make things worse, not better. When I have a sore lower back, for example, I apply moist heat for about 30 minutes. It helps my muscles relax, and as they relax, my pain level decreases.

There are two types of heat treatment. A heating pad or heat pack provides dry heat. Avoid putting dry heat directly on your skin. I wrap my heat packs in a pillowcase or apply them over a T-shirt. With dry heat, be mindful of the time elapsed. If you use a commercial product, follow the guidelines on the packaging.

Moist heat is administered with a steam towel or a soak in a bathtub or hot tub. I encourage you to experiment to see what works best for you. Heat packs and pads are generally more quick and convenient, but if I am feeling sore all over after rolling in Brazilian jiujitsu, sitting in a hot tub is more effective and relaxing.

Cold treatment can also take many forms—from ice cubes in a sealable plastic bag, to commercial ice packs, to soaking a sore ankle in a tub or bucket of ice water.

Icing an injury reduces blood flow, decreases inflammation, and quiets nerve endings (which decreases pain). You should ice a muscle or joint for only ten to fifteen minutes at a time—four or five times daily. Some doctors I know recommend longer icing sessions. Here is the rule of thumb I follow: When my ankle (or whatever) starts to go numb from the ice, it's time to take a break. As with too much heat, too much cold can cause tissue damage. That's why I follow my rule of thumb rather than the directions on a commercial ice pack. Once my skin goes numb, I might get a case of freezer burn without even knowing it.

Here are a couple of other distinctions between hot and cold treatments. I might use some moist, warm heat on my lower back before a workout or competition. It can relax a muscle and increase blood flow. However, I would not ice a sore ankle before a run. Ice makes joints stiff and decreases blood flow to an area. That's the last thing you need when you are about to exercise or compete.

If you suffer from arthritis, you might know that this condition can benefit from *both* treatments, depending on the kind of relief you seek. Heat can loosen stiff joints, while cold helps reduce swelling.

On the other hand, if you have circulatory issues, are diabetic, or have an injury that includes a cut or abrasion, check with a doctor before using heat or ice.

In fact, checking with a doctor or physical therapist is good general advice for all of us. This is especially true if you have suffered an injury that doesn't respond to treatment. For example, if I tweak my ankle on the basketball court and that ankle is still sore and swollen after 48 hours (despite icing and taking anti-inflammatories), I know it's time to make an appointment.

37

Finding a Gem of a Gym

I am writing this chapter in January, which happens to be my least favorite month to visit my local gym. It's always packed. It's hard to find a locker. I have to wait a long time for a weight machine or an exercise bike to free up.

As you might guess, more people join a gym in January than any other month. Thank you, New Year's resolutions! But many of these people don't stick around. According to the International Health, Racquet, and Sportsclub Association, the annual attrition rates for gyms is about 25 percent annually. I have worked with gyms with much higher rates than that—often more than 50 percent.

If reading this book has encouraged you to join or rejoin a gym, I congratulate you. Finding a well-equipped, well-staffed gym can be a huge factor in improving your overall health.

But how can you improve the chances that you will join a gym in January and still be showing up in August? It's all about finding the right facility for you. There are more than 32,000 gyms and health clubs in the United States alone, so finding the perfect one might take a little effort, but it's worth it. I'll offer a few tips. And even if you are already a gym member, please read this chapter. Maybe you will be encouraged to switch gyms or fitness clubs.

Go Local

Try to find a facility that is close to your home or workplace. The closer it is, the more likely you are to become a regular. Use Google Maps or some other tool to find gyms within a five-mile radius. Through my many years as a coach, athlete, and trainer, I have found a direct, inverse correlation between the distance traveled to a gym and the likelihood people become regulars. Most people won't drive more than 15 minutes or so. They start rationalizing: "Man, it's going to be 30 minutes round trip just to get there and back. And then I have to deal with finding a parking place and getting dressed and…"

Does this sound familiar?

> I have found a direct, inverse correlation between the distance traveled to a gym and the likelihood people become regulars.

Check Out the Prime-Time Schedule

If you tend to work out on your lunch break, don't visit a prospective gym on a quiet Sunday afternoon. The vibe might be completely different. More important, the equipment availability *will* be completely different. So visit that gym at lunchtime. If there is a waiting line at every exercise bike, or if there is simply no floor space at that midday exercise class, you might need to keep looking.

Think National

This tip might not apply if you don't travel much, but if you do, consider the big picture. Some chains have locations nationwide. Others, like the YMCA, offer "gym reciprocity" with other YMCAs around the country.

Seek Clean Machines

Some gyms bill themselves as muscle factories or fitness factories, but they can also be germ factories. In one study, researchers found 25 kinds of bacteria on a variety of fitness-center surfaces.[1]

Don't be afraid to ask the gym staff how often they clean the machines, bathrooms, and locker rooms—and *how* they clean them. Ideally, staff members should be wiping down the machines throughout

---

[1] Nabanita Mikherjee et al., "Diversity of Bacterial Communities of Fitness Center Surfaces in a U.S. Metropolitan Area," National Center for Biotechnology Information, December 3, 2014, https://www.ncbi.nlm.nih.gov/pmc/articles/PMC4276630/.

the day. Likewise, gym members should wipe down machines after using them. Look for dispensers of antiseptic wipes—and these receptacles should not always be empty. Also, I love seeing bottles of hand sanitizer strategically placed throughout a gym.

Ask About the Emergency Plan

No one heads to the gym with the thought of having a heart attack or some other emergency. But it happens. Ask if staff members are trained in CPR and general first aid. Is the facility equipped with an AED (automated external defibrillator)? These devices significantly improve a person's chance of surviving a cardiac incident. (By the way, you should ask this same question about your workplace.)

Check That Contract

If you search "complaints about gyms" online, expect "contracts" to be at or near the top of the list. Don't believe what the salesperson is promising you. Make sure those promises are backed up in writing. Does the contract require an automatic deduction from your bank account or credit card? Are you okay with that? And if you do go forward with your membership, check your bank or credit card statements carefully. Watch for the correct monthly charge and make sure no penalties or added fees have been tacked on.

While we are talking about contracts and fine print, make sure you know what happens if the club goes out of business or changes ownership. (This happens more often than one might think.)

One final note: If you sign a contract with a health club but then learn something that makes you regret that decision, you generally have from three to ten days to change your mind. (Laws about this vary from state to state.)

Watch for Signs of Good (or Bad) Management

Gyms are like a lot of other things in life: The little things can mean a lot. Is there a sign in the locker room prohibiting cell phone use? This shows that the management cares about your privacy.

Are there signs around the gym with messages like "Please watch your language" or "Please don't rest on the machines"? This shows that management cares about everyone's gym experience. This is important in an age when many people seem to go to the gym just to park themselves on a machine and text their friends for a half hour or so.

On a similar note, some gyms have private saunas or hot tubs connected to the men's and women's locker rooms. If so, there should be a sign indicating that swimwear should be worn in both areas. This is another "sign" of thoughtful management and the respect for members' privacy and comfort levels.

Put Your Money Where Your Muscles Are

If you have found a gym that you believe is right for you, think about putting some money down on some group personal training, a bonus exercise class, or some other option that will require regular attendance. Think of it as an accountability deposit. It's not just extra money to spend—it's a bit of extra protection for your investment.

Look Beyond the Bargains

Yes, there are good bargain gyms out there, but when it comes to fitness centers, you often get what you pay for. It's worth a few extra dollars a month for better equipment, a cleaner club, a more knowledgeable staff, and so on. One gym I really like has a bank of TVs in front of the cardio equipment. They broadcast a variety of shows and sporting events and provide health tips and reminders about gym rules and policies.

And here is another caveat about bargain gyms: If you think you're getting a steal of a deal at the gym, it is easier to justify failing to show up regularly—or at all.

Look for a Machine Mix

When you tour a gym, take careful note of the various machines. Are they all from one company or from multiple vendors? In other words, did the gym buy all its equipment from one vendor, perhaps because they got a good deal? Or did they source multiple options and pick the best of the best? My years as a competitor and trainer have shown me that one company might make a top-flight treadmill but subpar weight machines.

Along the same lines, ask when the equipment was purchased and how often it's upgraded.

One final note before we close this chapter. As you tour a prospective gym, note how many machines are broken or out of order. A well-managed gym will have a note on these machines, apologizing for the inconvenience and noting when the repair is expected to be completed.

If a note happens to be scrawled with marker on a torn sheet of paper (and half of the words are misspelled), that is *not* a sign of good management.

38

Find Your Sport

One of the best ways to stay active and healthy is to take up a sport or activity you can enjoy regularly.

I know this suggestion can sound intimidating, especially if you didn't participate in competitive sports in high school or college. But you don't have to be a hard-core competitor to take up a sport. You don't have to beat anybody or worry about someone defeating you. Instead, focus on learning something new and enjoyable or reacquainting yourself with a sport or activity you once enjoyed.

> You don't have to be a hard-core competitor to take up a sport. You don't have to beat anybody or worry about someone defeating you. Instead, focus on learning something new and enjoyable or reacquainting yourself with a sport or activity you once enjoyed.

It could be as simple as heading out the door and seeing how far you can run. Your goal could be to double that distance in a month or two.

If you need a few ideas or suggestions, here is a list of some of the sports stuff I have tried (or retried) since I turned 18.

surfing	kayaking
snowboarding	swimming
snow-skiing	strongman competitions
water-skiing	jiujitsu
skateboarding	Olympic-style weight lifting
in-line skating	powerlifting

triathlons	shot put
mountain biking	discus
climbing (mountains, rock, and ice)	running (various distances)
basketball	obstacle courses
rugby	longboarding
kettlebells	hiking

This list is just off the top of my head. I am probably leaving something out, but you get the idea. I am sharing this list not to show off, but to encourage you to try something—and to be willing to fail. Like me, you might find that you stink at some sports. But try to have fun with it and learn from the experience.

As I look at my list, I can assure you that I was *not* proficient at all these sports and activities. In fact, I was not even decent at many of them. But I didn't let that stop me from trying each one at least a few times. I encourage you to give yourself a chance. Think about your life—and not just your sporting life. Think about the stuff that eventually got easier the more you learned and the more you tried.

Remember the first time you drove a car? Were you an expert the first time you settled in behind the wheel? I certainly wasn't. But like me, I bet you consider yourself an expert driver now.

In high school, I participated in football, basketball, and track and field. In football, I was being recruited by some major NCAA Division 1 schools before an injury ended my career.

Today, my "major" sport is Brazilian jiujitsu—a new venture for me. I am only a blue belt right now (just the second of the five belts you can earn), but I am making progress. I moved out of my comfort zone and had to start from scratch, but I am enjoying the process.

People have told me, "It's easy for you to promote sports participation. You're a competitive athlete. I can barely walk."

My response? "Then 'barely walk' as much as you can. Try to increase your distance a little bit at a time. Don't try to be me—or anyone else. Just be the best *you* you can be."

Exercise is something our bodies were meant to do. We are not meant to be sedentary. Regular movement (whatever kind of movement you can do) is so good for you physically, mentally, and spiritually. I know an older gentleman who cannot get around without a walker. His initial goal was to simply cover the distance from his front door to his mailbox at the end of the driveway. After a few weeks of trying, he was making four or five round trips every day.

I strongly believe that physical activity is as effective as medication, if not more so, in treating some kinds of depression. Whatever your go-to sport or activity, it will help you lose fat and keep it off. It will keep you strong and limber. And it will make your brain work better. (By the way, for great insights on how your brain health connects to your overall health and fitness, I recommend the book *60 Ways to Keep Your Brain Sharp* by Bonnie Sparrman.)

As you consider your sport options, go with what fits you and your lifestyle best. And of course, if you have any health challenges, get recommendations from a medical professional. But please try something! Find some buddies for a regular game of pickup basketball or H-O-R-S-E. Start a walking club at work. Take a fitness class or a dance class. And these classes don't have to be intense or intimidating. Some gyms offer "Be Fit While You Sit" classes, where most of the exercises can be done from a chair.

Start playing golf with friends once a week. If some of them bail, that's okay. You can keep at it. If you can't challenge each other, you can still challenge yourself. It's never too late to try. Here is something I have observed over the years—people who participated in a sport or regular athletic activity in midlife were much more likely to be active and healthy when they entered their so-called golden years.

Your sport doesn't have to be high intensity or high impact. I think of a sport like Ping-Pong. It improves your fine motor skills, hand-eye coordination, flexibility, balance, and lateral movement. And when was the last time you heard of someone being sidelined by a Ping-Pong-related injury?

When selecting your sport, go with what you enjoy (or think you might enjoy). Don't go with what is trendy or has the coolest gear. Choose what your body can tolerate. (You want something that will challenge you but not crush you.) Over the long haul, you won't stick with something you hate. The same goes for something that is a bad fit for you based on age, temperament, injury history, and so on.

One reason I love sports and organized activities is that they keep us from slacking off. If I am by myself in the gym, I might be tempted to get sloppy or to cut my workout short if I am feeling tired or lazy. But if I am playing basketball with some friends on open gym night or in the church basketball league, I've got to keep up.

If you are in your forties or beyond, you might not be able to indulge your number one choice for sports. I have several friends who love full-court, full-speed basketball, but some of them have endured significant knee injuries or foot injuries. Their bodies simply won't tolerate an hour of full-court running and jumping. But they have found other outlets. A couple of them play tennis. Another one still plays a little basketball, but in the form of H-O-R-S-E and Around the World.

Whatever sport you choose, I recommend supplementing it with stretching, yoga, and other exercises that build muscle, core strength, and flexibility. This way, you will improve your game and reduce your risk of injury—on the court, field, or wherever.

Consider teaming up with some old friends or making some new ones. You will probably find that this combination of fitness and fellowship reduces stress and keeps you motivated.

As we close this chapter, here are my top-five tips to help you get the most out of your sports participation.

1. *Eat smart.* You will find that participating in a sport requires high-quality fuel. Playing a sport regularly motivates me to eat more thoughtfully.
2. *Hydrate.* Don't wait until ten minutes before a volleyball match or basketball game to start gulping water. Hydration should be

a daily habit, especially on game day and the days leading up to it.

3. *Enlist a friend.* You are more likely to keep at it if you enjoy the people you compete with—and even against. It's nice knowing that I'll get some good-natured teasing from the guys at my MMA gym if I miss a workout.

4. *Know your limits.* If you go too hard or too long, you risk injury. Take a break if you need to. Let someone sub in for you during the basketball game. Don't try to be the first to finish every training run with your running group.

5. *Keep things in perspective.* Remember, you are now playing for fun and fitness; you aren't trying to impress pro scouts. The score of your community softball league game will not appear on the front page of the sports section. If you get tossed out of a church league basketball game for arguing with the volunteer referee, that's a good sign you've lost your sense of perspective.

39

Getting the Work Done 101

The future is purchased by the present.
Samuel Johnson

The good news: If you're reading this book, you're already on your way to becoming a healthier, happier person.

The not-so-good news: This new, healthier phase of your life is probably going to involve lots of learning, priority balancing, and schedule making.

But here's more good news: The challenges ahead of you can be easier to manage than those of your recent past. You can build on the knowledge you've accumulated so far, and you can implement *what* you've learned about *how* you learn as you strive to eat better, exercise more, and generally take better care of yourself.

Allow me to explain that last statement. People learn in different ways. Some learn best by reading, others by hearing or seeing, and still others by doing. What about you? Can you read a chapter of a book and retain almost everything? Or do you often have to pore over the same page two or three times before the words start to make an imprint on your brain?

In a similar vein, are you one of those people who can read a set of directions and then deftly assemble a piece of furniture or hook up a sound system? Or maybe the written directions read like Sanskrit to you, but if you watch someone *demonstrating* a skill, you can pick it up almost immediately. (This is why a personal trainer can be such an asset to many people who want to learn new exercises.)

You get the point. As you strive to be a healthier person, play to your strengths. If you learn best by hearing, for example, listen to health-related podcasts during your morning commute or while you speed walk on the treadmill.

If the written word is your thing, your best bet might be a good old-fashioned session of hitting the books, magazines, or websites. I like to grab a fitness or health magazine at the gym and read a few articles while I'm on an exercise bike. And I eagerly await the next fitness book by authors I respect and look up to.

And you might improve your learning prowess even further by writing down (or typing) key facts or formulas you need to know. This added step reinforces learning as information passes from your eyes to your brain to your hands and then through the system again as you read what you just committed to paper (or a computer screen).

Here's another tip for making your learning time more effective: Control your environment. Just as people have different preferred learning methods, they also vary when it comes to work settings. If you're easily distracted, the local coffee shop—with its hissing espresso machines, chatting customers, and busy baristas—might dangle too many distractions that can pull your attention away from what you're reading.

On the other hand, crazy as it might sound, some people find silence intimidating and stifling. These people would much rather read a new fitness bestseller in that noisy coffee shop than on an isolated back porch.

As with learning styles, you might need to experiment with environments to find your sweet spot. But eventually it will become clear where you're most effective—and least frustrated and distracted. The important thing is to give yourself permission to find out what works for you. And don't be afraid to ask a personal trainer, nutritionist, or fitness coach to accommodate your optimum learning or workout style. A good leader should be cool with helping you succeed rather than enforcing rules for the sake of rules. The same thing goes for your personal physician.

Don't be afraid to ask a personal trainer, nutritionist,
or fitness coach to accommodate your optimum
learning or workout style.

With what we have learned about learning styles and environments in mind, I want to close this chapter by offering my "Three Simple Rules for Getting Stuff Done."

Back Off!

In this case, "back off" means to create a back-off schedule for whatever you're working on. Start with the due date and then—working backward from that date to the present—set a series of progressive goals and intermediate deadlines that will help you meet that big final deadline. I know someone who recently competed in the Boston Marathon, and I was impressed by how strategic and detailed their training schedule was. A back-off schedule helps avoid surprises and is a great tool for keeping you on task and monitoring your progress. (This book wouldn't exist if not for its own back-off schedule.)

Break It Down

"How do you eat an elephant?" the famous theoretical question goes. The answer? "One bite at a time." If you yearn to run your first marathon someday, consider starting with a 5K (3.1 miles). If that goes well, move up to a 5-miler or a 10K. I am using a similar approach as I write this book. I didn't just sit down one day and crank out this chapter. Instead, this was my approach:

- Write an outline.
- Research.
- Write intro and first three paragraphs.
- Finish main chapter and begin "Three Simple Rules" closer.
- Finish "Three Simple Rules" closer.
- Edit and fact-check.

Get Help

Suffering in silence might be noble, but it won't help you get work done or prepare for a big race, tennis match, mountain hike, or other fitness challenge. If you're struggling, tell somebody. Seek help from a friend. Make a doctor's appointment if you need to. If you have been struggling to get through workouts lately or you've noticed dramatic changes in your weight, something might be up. Perhaps it's a virus. Perhaps you have developed a food allergy. Whatever the case, this is *your* health and well-being at stake. If you have a concern or fear, it's worth getting checked out. You're worth it.

40

Execute Your Excuses

As we approach the end of part 2, I thank you and compliment you for sticking with me so far. Parts 1 and 2 contain a lot of information to take in. There is a good reason for that. It takes time and effort to make any significant changes in life, but you are worth it. If there is one bit of self-talk I'd like you to glean from this book, that's it—"I am worth it."

When you have to get up earlier in the morning, either to eat a good breakfast or go for an early run, tell yourself, "I'm worth it." When you pass on the offer to go out for drinks and appetizers with coworkers, remind yourself, "I am worth it."

In time, you will find that valuing yourself and your health will help you be more conscientious and consistent when buying groceries or eating out. These days, I find myself buying more salads and opting for grilled meat instead of the breaded and fried stuff. Whenever I am tempted to consume something I know I really shouldn't, I remind myself of how hard I have worked, how much progress I have made.

And when I do backslide (yes, it happens), I look at it as an aberration. It's a fluke, not the first step down a long and destructive road.

Excuses abound when it comes to exercise as well. "I forgot to pack my gym clothes today" or "I don't really have the right shoes for basketball, and that's what I really wanted to do today."

I tried to excuse-proof myself by simply committing to always being ready. I keep a go-bag in my car. I make sure it has at least a pair of shorts, a T-shirt, and my backup pair of tennis shoes. I want to be ready to take advantage of any downtime that might pop up. In a similar vein, I know lots of people who keep a pair of walking shoes at work.

Also, when I travel, I wear walking shoes or athletic shoes as a rule. If my flight is delayed (which happens *all* the time), I take a walk around the airport. Sometimes, the delay is so significant that I meet my daily one-hour walking goal while waiting to board.

> When I travel, I wear walking shoes or athletic shoes as a rule.
> If my flight is delayed (which happens *all* the time),
> I take a walk around the airport.

What about those delays that happen after you are already in your airline seat? Well, do what you can. Do a few stretches and deep-breathing routines. And you can do some exercises in an airplane seat without injuring your seatmates. Isometrics are one option, but I also like to do some ankle rotations, calf raises, and bent-leg raises.

While we are on the subject of travel, I should point out another health-sabotaging problem with business trips. Some people rationalize, "I'm going to be eating mostly fast food this week, so why even bother trying to be healthy?"

Wrong. There is such a thing as healthful fast food these days. Even the burger places have some decent options. Look for the "heart healthy" section of the menu. If you use a service like Grubhub, you can modify your order in the "notes" section. For example, I often order a grilled chicken sandwich with the sauce on the side. I have found that my order is less likely to get messed up if I order the sauce, gravy, or dressing on the side rather than ordering my entrée without it. (That's also true when I order at a restaurant. Go figure.)

Guess what? Sometimes I still find sauce on my chicken sandwich. I scrape off all the gunk, toss the bun, and eat my chicken with a knife and fork.

Yes, sometimes eating right and exercising faithfully can be challenging. But I deal with the frustration and make no excuses. Because I am worth it. So are you.

41

Don't Try to Out-Train a Bad Diet!

I wasn't sure if I should put this chapter in the diet section or the exercise section. I chose the latter, but this concept is so important, I was tempted to put it in both sections!

I wish I had a dollar for every time I have told someone, "You can't out-train a bad diet." It's true, of course, but you might not believe how many people think that a hard workout covers a multitude of dietary sins. It doesn't. There are about 500 calories in a large frozen mocha coffee drink. You can drink one in ten minutes or so, but it can take an hour of hard work to burn those calories.

Health and training professionals generally agree that good health is 70 percent diet and 30 percent exercise. This ratio alone should show the importance of a healthy approach to eating.

> Health and training professionals generally agree that good health is 70 percent diet and 30 percent exercise.

But how many times have you heard someone say, "I worked out today, so I can have this big piece of chocolate cake" or "I can eat the donuts in the office because I'm going to run after work." It's such an easy trap to fall into. You crush your workout at the gym but reward yourself by overindulging.

Let me be clear (again). If you are striving to lose weight, you need to live in Calorie Deficit Land. As we've seen, losing weight and staying healthy involves some simple math. Let's say you set a goal to lose one pound a week. That means your weekly calorie deficit number needs to be about 3,500 calories. That's seven Frappuccinos (if you like your coffee drinks sweet and frozen).

Let's take this math further. To burn 3,500 calories, you need to work out seven days a week for about an hour and a half every day, depending on the type of activity. Most of us simply don't have that kind of time. We might get injured or hit the wall if we went this hard with no days for rest and recovery.

Indeed, it's almost impossible, especially for those of us who have busy lives and don't want to spend all our discretionary time at the gym.

A guy recently told me, "I worked out regularly this week, and I ate great too. I only cheated over the weekend when I treated myself to a cheeseburger, fries, soda, and a dessert. So I think I'm going to like my numbers next time I step on the scale."

I explained to this guy that his single fast-food meal probably added up to 2,000 calories, if not more. That is a whole day's worth of calories based on a sensible diet. For this guy, about 40 years old and in decent shape, one hour of weight training plus a half hour of cardio burns about 700 calories. That is only about one-third of the calories in his single meal!

I wrote down the key numbers and asked him, "Can you see why bad dieting outweighs good training almost every time?"

And even if you don't do the cheat meal thing, how many of us have a heavily sweetened coffee drink in the morning? How many of us have a beer or two after work once or twice a week? Just a few of these smaller indulgences put us over the top when it comes to calories—and these are *empty* calories.

This is where terms like "yo-yo dieting" or "roller-coaster dieting" come from. You are working out regularly and eating healthfully most of the time. You reward yourself by overindulging. You feel guilty about this and work out even harder. But this can lead to more rewards or justifications at the fast-food counter, food truck, or donut shop. Can you see the problem with the concept of cheat meals or cheat days?

One day I was on a long drive and pulled into a truck stop. A huge cinnamon roll caught my eye when I walked through the door. The pastry looked tempting, but I did a quick reality check. I estimated the roll's calorie content at about 500. I know how much effort it takes to burn 500 calories, and on this trip, I didn't have time to burn that many. I reminded myself that the human body can store thousands of calories as fat. Then I ate a piece of fresh fruit and drank water instead.

Now, if this trip had included the chance for some full-court basketball with friends or a couple of long runs, I *might* have chosen differently. The key was making a thoughtful decision, looking at the big caloric picture, and not acting on impulse.

I encourage you to learn and practice balance. Embrace a healthy lifestyle. Lean into it, as they say. Yes, it's okay to have the occasional cheat day, but if you look at health as a lifestyle, you will find that your taste buds change. Your mindset changes. I know people who get a charge out of *cheating* on their cheat day.

A buddy recently told me, "I was going to have a milkshake on Saturday, but I decided to have a fruit and veggie smoothie instead. And with this kind of 'cheating,' I feel good, not guilty!"

If you broaden your perspective, your deep-fried cravings won't haunt you as often. And when they do poke up their heads like prairie dogs, you will have gained power over them.

Your willpower will be rewarded. You will appreciate how far you have come, and you will see no good reason to start taking steps backward.

Part 3

Rest, Recover, Recharge

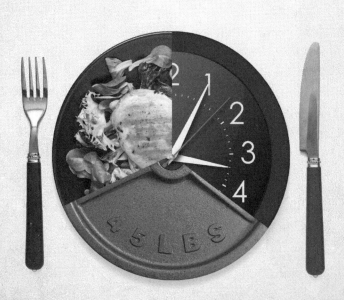

42

Make the Necessary Recovery Efforts

Sometimes the effort to stay healthy and fit takes its toll. I know the feeling. Especially if you are 40 or over, as I am, you might find that it takes several days for you to feel rested and not sore after a hard workout, tennis match, or long hike. It makes you less likely to hit the gym, the pool, or the running trail again. I have seen people get off to a fast start with a fitness program but then hit the wall due to a combination of soreness and sluggishness.

That's why I caution the people I work with to avoid overtraining. It can be tempting to push, push, push to get results faster. But you must train smart and give your body a chance to recover as you go.

If you find yourself sore and tired after crushing a workout but you really don't want to interrupt your schedule, go ahead and keep training but reduce the time or the amount of weight resistance. Or both.

Eventually, your body will learn to adapt. When I say it's okay to back off on the intensity, I am not saying that you should stop improving or that you should never put more weight on the bar. But I do advise taking more time to build up to the next level. This has an added benefit. You can perfect your form and technique as you recover a bit. This prevents injury and ensures you are working the muscles you intend to work. I have seen people develop all kinds of bad habits, such as bouncing the bench-press bar off their chests or arching their backs or rolling back and forth instead of doing an actual sit-up.

Also, focus on nutrition. Within the first half hour or so after your weight session, for example, consume about 20 grams of high-quality protein (whey protein powder or pea protein, for example). Add some fast-absorbing carbs as well. They help maximize your muscle recovery through increased protein synthesis. I like low-sugar sports drinks with electrolytes too. They help replenish your glycogen stores in addition to restoring your electrolyte balance.

And please, try to get at least seven to nine hours of sleep nightly. (I hit this theme often for very good reasons.) Don't "find time" to sleep. *Make* time. I offer this same advice for exercise, eating right, and so on. As much as possible, go to sleep at the same time every night.

> Try to get seven to nine hours of sleep nightly.
> Don't "find time" to sleep. *Make* time.

I realize this is not always possible. Some of us have crazy work schedules, and I have some friends who travel with their kids' sports teams for months at a time. There is almost no way for them to keep any kind of reliable schedule.

For people like this, I emphasize that all of one's sleep does not have to come at night. Grab a 30-minute nap when you can. Sleep on the plane. Sleep in the car—if you aren't the one driving!

As I close this chapter, I emphasize that sleep is not only vital as you recover and recharge after hard workouts; it's also key to your overall health. Some people brag about being able to perform just fine on three or four hours of sleep. However, most of us need between seven and nine hours of sleep every night. If we go too long without adequate sleep, we slip into a "sleep debt." A chronic lack of sleep has been linked to a variety of problems, including obesity, high blood pressure, and mood swings. What's more, operating in sleep debt can affect your productivity on the job and even your ability to drive a vehicle safely.

43

Focus on the "Rest" of Your Story

As a member of the human race, you need to rest occasionally. You may be young and have lots to do. Perhaps you have plenty of adrenaline—and maybe plenty of Red Bull—flowing through your veins, and you feel indestructible, indefatigable.

You still need to chill sometimes. Take time to recover physically, emotionally, and spiritually from life's demands—including the demands associated with your quest for better health. You need time to take stock of where you've been, where you are, and where you are headed. You need quiet, reflective, and restful moments—away from stress, work or assignments, and to-do lists. You need to take the time to be a friend, a parent, a spouse, a son or daughter, a brother or sister, a thoughtful being.

It's ironic that the animal kingdom has figured out this principle, but many of the so-called more advanced creatures haven't. Japan's snow monkeys, for example, work hard just to stay alive in their frigid habitat. They must climb high mountains continuously as they search for food. But they take frequent breaks to rest and renew themselves and even monkey around a little. They seem to have an innate understanding that all work and no play leads to exhaustion—and maybe extinction.

Contrast the monkeys with some of Japan's human workers who have literally worked themselves to death. I am not kidding about this. Some have dropped dead at their desks. The drive for performance—exemplified not only by output but also by hours put in—permeates the Japanese work culture. This tragic syndrome has become so prevalent that it's been given its own name—*karoshi*.

Yes, it's possible to become so obsessed with work, school, or even fitness activities that you ignore your body's physical and mental signals that it needs rest and replenishment. It's not wise to disregard those signals. Various studies reveal that those who fail to recharge their mental and physical batteries are more susceptible to illness and stress-related problems, such as ulcers, and to mistakes on the job. Rest can help you avoid such perils.

Additionally, in resting you will find the time and the right frame of mind to contemplate the wonders of life. And you can gather the energy to live your life to the fullest.

There's no question—you need rest to be at your best. But rest can be elusive. How can you fit some downtime into an already-crowded life? Here are a few tips.

First, build rest time into your daily schedule. Let's face it, if you're like most people (including me), that's the only way to ensure balance in your life. And it's okay to be a bit selfish, a bit inflexible about this rest time. If you aren't, something else will crowd it out. Take a regular ten-minute head-clearing walk after lunch or at break time on the job. Or read a book for pleasure, not as a work or school assignment. Or just use those minutes as chill time. One businessperson I know goes to his car every afternoon, reclines his seat, and grabs a 15-minute power nap.

Another great way to take a load off is to pursue interests and hobbies that differ from what you do on the job. And in this case, adopting a favorite TV show, web series, or podcast can count as an interest. This strategy can help you engage and feed your brain and body in a way that your job does not. At the same time, it will give those often-used job-related parts a needed respite.

Finally, get adequate sleep at night. This advice bears repeating. Your body needs it. Your mind needs it. Sure, you might be able to get more work done if you sleep fewer hours each night, but at what cost? Turn off the TV at the appropriate time. Enough with the texting and posting. Close the laptop. Sleep.

To be at your best, to be healthy, to be a well-rounded person, to fully and truly enjoy life, you must find the time to rest your body, mind, and spirit. Think of all the extra hours you spend working and then worrying about what's going on at work. Think of what that time could mean to your family, your friends, your spiritual life, and your well-being.

Beware of the barrenness of an overcrowded life.

AMERICAN PROVERB

44

Enjoy Some Rare Air

Consider this: Oxygen is life. Without breath, we are not alive. My EMT buddies tell me that restoring the ability to breathe is the first priority for saving and preserving life. It's no accident that the book of Genesis speaks of humanity becoming alive when God breathed the breath of life into us.

This might seem like a weird question, but do you breathe enough? Most people don't. They breathe too quickly and too shallowly. I see it every day. And people breathe too much indoor air—*recycled* indoor air. Do you know how many dead skin particles are floating around the air in your workplace or local mall? Google that and see if you aren't inspired to get outside more for some fresh air.

Most people simply do not get enough of the miraculous exchange: The pure, life-giving oxygen coming in and the carbon dioxide and toxins going out.

Did you know that becoming more aware of your breathing and breathing more slowly and deeply can lower your stress level and make you healthier? It's true.

> Becoming more aware of your breathing and
> breathing more slowly and deeply can lower your
> stress level and make you healthier.

If you can, stop reading right now and go outside for an oxygen supplement. When you get out there, take seven or eight big breaths. Nice and slow. Relax and taaake your tiiime…try to feel that fresh air gracing your trillions of cells. You are alive! You are alive because God gave you your very breath. He did that because he loves you.

Next, breathe in and hold in that air gratefully. Blow it out, grateful for the next wonderful breath waiting for you.

I hope that when you have completed this task, you will feel different. I hope you are glad you took the time to get beyond the walls and truly breathe.

And if you are tempted to skip this exercise with the intention that you'll do it later, please don't wait. (Unless you are reading this book on an airplane, of course. In that case, you are excused until you are safely outside the terminal.)

Here's what you accomplish with all that breathing and why it is awesome.

According to our best science, you have just spread a calming effect throughout your entire nervous system. You have released tension in your muscles and lowered your blood pressure. You also triggered positive results in your brain, digestive system, lymph system, and immune system.

Breathing in a slow, controlled, intentional manner changes the response of your body's autonomic nervous system, which (without your knowledge) controls other systems, including digestion and circulation. Breathing is linked to these systems. And it is impossible to relax these without breathing more slowly and taking in more oxygen. It is also impossible to breathe in this manner and fail to reap the benefits I have just described. When you focus on and control your breathing, you are setting off automatic positive effects throughout your body.

And we haven't even touched on what you are doing for your mind. Because your mind and body are linked, there is a calming effect on your mind as your body relaxes. We know this is true because we have discovered neurochemicals and the parasympathetic branch of the nervous system. Neurochemicals send signals that tell your body how to feel. Basically, when you breathe this way, your brain gets a message that all is well, and your body responds involuntarily.

In a recent study of people with major depression, after 12 weeks of regular coherent breathing (in this case, in a type of yoga class), the participants showed a significant increase in gamma-aminobutyric acid, a brain chemical associated with calming and antianxiety effects. Additionally, participants reported that their anxiety and depressive symptoms decreased![1]

What does all this science mean? Slow, deep, intentional breathing is one of the very best things you can do for your body and mind. And it will reduce the negative effects of stress on your body. Let all of this breathe for a while. Then let *yourself* breathe.

---

[1] National Institutes of Health, National Center for Complementary and Integrative Health, "Relaxation Techniques for Health," May 2016, https://nccih.nih.gov/health/stress/relaxation.htm#hed1.

45

Life Moving Too Fast?
Time to Techno-Fast

You have probably heard the term "technology fast" (or "techno-fast"), but have you ever tried it? Most of us wouldn't know what to do without our mobile devices, but how many of us have considered what all the screen-based technology is doing to us?

In his thought-provoking (and bestselling) book *The Shallows: What the Internet Is Doing to Our Brains*, Nicholas Carr explores some research indicating that technology is changing the "wiring" of our brains. Specifically, we are losing the ability to "deep read," to sit alone without distractions and truly contemplate and experience the magic of a book. We are losing our ability to focus. Think about the implications of this for your Bible study time, for example. Think about how long it's been since you had the amazing and wonderful experience of getting lost in a good book, including the Good Book.

I admit, the first time someone suggested that my smartphone and I needed some time apart, I thought, "No way. I can't get through the day without my phone."

But then I thought some more and wondered how I had gotten to the point where I couldn't survive without a little rectangle of technology that didn't even exist 20 years ago. I thought back to those days from my early twenties. I didn't have an internet-enabled device that accompanied me everywhere I went. I didn't stay perpetually connected to hundreds of people every second of the day. I didn't get pictures of their every meal and snack. I didn't know what music they were all listening to (right now!) on Spotify. I didn't see the costumes they were putting on their cats. And I survived!

Today, it's different. We have all been "left to our own devices," and we are less peaceful and more stressed out than ever. If our tablets, smartphones, smart watches, and so on truly contain all the answers to peace and happiness, why are we all on meds to combat depression and anxiety?

As technology early adaptors, we are more connected than ever, but as human beings, we are less connected than ever. We have more casual, surface relationships than any generation in history, but our deepest and most important relationships are suffering. How many times have you seen two people on a date at a restaurant staring at their smartphones? I have seen the same thing with married couples and moms and dads with their kids—kids as young as seven or eight.

> We have more casual, surface relationships than
> any generation in history, but our deepest and most
> important relationships are suffering.

We are less aware of the important people in our lives. We are less aware of ourselves.

So *now* can I suggest a techno-fast to you?

And please don't panic. A techno-fast doesn't have to be painful. It doesn't have to be forever. Here are a few suggestions I encourage you to consider.

Go for a walk and leave your smartphone at home. On purpose. While you're outside, you can notice that the earth is still spinning, and life as we know it has not ended. In fact, you'll notice all kinds of remarkable things when not staring down at a screen.

Put your phone away (out of sight) when in the presence of your loved ones. You will notice better face-to-face interaction (you know, the way we were made to interact). This works best when you ask those loved ones to do the same. If this seems overwhelming, pick a time to do it. Some families reserve this policy for dinner or all mealtimes. The Love and Logic Institute started a wonderful trend called Phone Down Friday (#PhoneDownFriday, #PDF), in which a day of the week (it doesn't have to be Friday, of course) is reserved for paying more attention to loved ones' faces and less attention to screens and devices. They even give parents a great line to use with their kids: "Time with you is important, so I'm putting my phone away while we're talking. Thank you for doing the same."

Go for a hike or nature walk and (gulp) don't bring your phone. Of course, you need to be smart about this. You don't want to embark on a long trek in the wilderness with no lifeline if something goes awry. But you can use safeguards, such as walking with someone or choosing a familiar and well-traveled area. You could also let someone know where you are going and how long you plan to be hiking or walking. In fact, you can even bring your device but turn it off and keep it zipped in a pocket.

While you are at work or at home, set a timer and see how long you can go without looking at your device. When you look, stop the timer. Now try to beat your record.

Pick a time of day (or maybe specific days of the week) devoted to returning emails and texts. This can be a long-term solution, as it will start to train people about the best times to contact or interact with you electronically. If the demands of your job don't allow for this approach, you can still target occasional days or times when you will be offline.

A book editor I know will send out occasional emails like this: "I will be immersed in book proposals all day tomorrow. I won't be checking emails or answering texts during this time." Other people I know will announce they are taking a break from social media for a while. (Some people give it up for Lent.) This way, no one will worry that you've dropped off the face of the earth—and they won't keep private messaging you with updates on their cat's digestive issues. When I announce a techno-fast like this, I challenge my friends and family to "go and do likewise."

Experiment with apps and settings that notify people you are unavailable (because you are driving, for example). I really like the concept of using technology to wean ourselves *off* technology.

46

Seek Inspiration

I know people who believe they are doomed to the same fate as their parents, grandparents, or other relatives. People have told me, "I know I'm going to get diabetes because almost everyone in my family has it."

I tell them, "Don't accept genetics as your fate. You have no idea what you can accomplish unless you try. Besides, this might *not* be a genetic thing."

For example, if I ate the way my former in-laws ate (we met them back in chapter 14), I would be overweight. And I would probably be prediabetic too. But I eat to keep my blood sugar levels normal. I eat to prevent disease and inflammation. I eat and exercise the way people I respect do.

When I was working in Afghanistan, I met a guy named Kyle. He was a living, breathing fitness model. He had six-pack abs, and his arms looked like they were about to burst free of whatever shirt was trying to contain them.

As I got to know him better, Kyle told me he was chubby as a kid. He got tired of being teased and being unable to perform at his physical best. He wanted something better for himself. This desire inspired him to start eating healthfully and exercising like a madman.

During this tour of duty in Afghanistan, I lived with Kyle 24/7. I saw how hard he worked to keep himself in shape. He was what people call a health nut. Another of our coworkers, Bill, would point at Kyle and say, "I wish I looked like you, but I don't have the genetics for it. I bet you don't even have to work that hard to look like you do."

I asked Bill what kind of diet and exercise regimen he practiced. He said he'd never really tried. "Then how do you know how you might look?" I asked him. I nodded toward Kyle, and asked Bill, "Do you know it took Kyle more than 12 years of hard work to get where he is today?"

I don't accept excuses. They give people an easy out and rob them of what they could be. When people start giving me excuses, I quote Zig Ziglar: "You have to change your stinkin' thinkin'!"

One of the best ways to overcome that kind of thinking is to surround yourself with mentors and people who inspire and support you. If you can afford it, consider hiring a personal trainer, even if it's just a short-term thing. A trainer can help you set realistic goals and custom design a fitness plan for you. Or find a workout buddy or two so you can encourage and support each other.

Read books, blogs, and articles that inspire you. Seek inspiration wherever you can find it. I often get all the inspiration I need from looking in the mirror. When I do this, I do more than assess my physical appearance. I ask myself if I am truly being all I can be. I ask myself if I am being the kind of person my kids will look up to.

One of the reasons I love to encourage people to develop self-discipline about their health is that self-discipline spills over into all areas of life—your job, your relationships, your educational pursuits, your spiritual life. Some of the fittest people I know are also at the top of their games in their career, in their marriages, and as parents.

> We should accept who God made us to be,
> but we should also strive to become the best
> possible version of who God made us to be.

I am not saying everyone should strive to look like Kyle. But we should be doers, not complainers. Yes, we should accept who God made us to be, but we should also strive to become the best possible version of who God made us to be.

Ignoring our health is a fast track to devolving into the worst we can be. So be confident in your potential. Be a doer. Become the kind of person your spouse wants you to be, or the kind of person a best friend wants you to be. If you are a parent, you should strive to be the kind of person you want your kids to become someday. Who wouldn't be inspired by that?

Choosing Life

Life can be all about choices. To be more intentional about finding peace and seeking inspiration, consider some of these choices:

outdoors versus indoors

simple versus complicated

park far away and walk versus fight for a close spot

fresh food versus junk food

water versus soda or alcohol

listening versus ranting

slowness or stillness versus hurry

thankfulness versus covetousness and want

appreciating versus worrying

reading versus watching junk TV

meditation versus playing video games

prayer versus junk social media

In other words, take your eyes off what the world is doing and turn your thoughts inward—and upward.

47

Seek Solitude, Not Isolation

One of the keys to recovering from a hard workout (or just the stress of life) is finding solitude. Even extroverts need some alone time to recharge themselves mentally, physically, and spiritually.

I want to draw a distinction between solitude and isolation. In today's world, unfortunately, we get plenty of isolation. As you might know, isolation doesn't necessarily equal being alone. I have friends who tell me how isolated they feel during their work commute even though they are surrounded by dozens of other vehicles. I know many others who feel isolated on their electronic devices. It's ironic that the term "connection" is used with our phones, tablets, and computers, but we aren't truly connected on a meaningful, personal level.

Electronic stimulation does not equal deep friendship or deep fellowship. Staring at a screen for hours a day does not provide solitude. It's not even an effective escape from stress. We humans were not made to connect with each other this way. We were crafted as relational creatures. We need truly personal, face-to-face communication.

I have friends and relatives who interact well when they encounter a baby—especially if they are related to that baby. They make eye contact. They smile. They coo and let the baby grasp their finger or tug on their hair. This is foundational communication. This is how humans can relate to one another, even when one of those humans cannot even speak yet. But in the adult world, the human smile has been replaced by an emoji. The laugh has been replaced by a GIF of a chuckling cartoon character.

The human smile has been replaced by an emoji. The laugh has been replaced by a GIF of a chuckling cartoon character.

What does all this have to do with solitude? I will explain. We often think of solitude as alone time, and sometimes we all need that. It can be relaxing and freeing to find some solitary time to think deeply, to reflect, to pray. However, I encourage you to seek solitude *with* another person (or small group of people) from time to time. This might be with your spouse—just the two of you getting away from the world's noise. It can be a few buddies going on a camping excursion. It can be a mother and daughter road trip, or a grandpa and grandkid fishing adventure. Sometimes, truly connecting with another person helps us get more in touch with ourselves.

This brings us to another aspect of solitude—movement. We were made to move, and we don't move enough, especially when it comes to being outdoors. I get frustrated when I see so many people living in a way that ignores the way we were made. That's why I love it when I see family members and friends heading out into nature. This provides the peace that comes from spending restorative, soul-strengthening time with those we love *and* experiencing the beauty and power of nature, the displays of God's awesomeness.

I can promise you that if you live in a way that is more in touch with how you are created, you will be more in touch with your Creator. It's all about balance. Just as there is a time for rest and a time for activity, there is also a time for aloneness and a time for community.

48

Know When to Call It a Night

*Come to me, all you who are weary and
burdened, and I will give you rest.*
MATTHEW 11:28

We have talked about rest and recovery in the context of exercise and fitness. But did you know that 164 million Americans have sleep troubles? That's more than half of the adult population.[1] Maybe you're one of them. Most of us need seven to nine hours of sleep nightly, and coming up short hits us where we hurt. Our memories aren't as sharp. Our skin doesn't get the time it needs to repair and rejuvenate itself. Our bodies tend to store more fat. Sleep deprivation has also been linked to high blood pressure, diabetes, depression, and even heightened mortality rates.

However, I have good news. You can take all the woes above and turn them upside down by improving your sleep habits.

Insomnia is typically categorized as either short-term or chronic. Short-term insomnia causes are things like jet lag, the birth of a new baby, or a new residence with its requisite new noises and sleep interrupters. Chronic sleep disorders tend to be those that last a month or more, resulting from such causes as apnea (breathing problems), depression, or a neurological disorder, such as restless legs syndrome.

Treatment choices abound for those with all kinds of sleeping problems. There are non-habit-forming, over-the-counter sleep aids as well as alternatives, like biofeedback or prescription medication.

[1] "Why Americans Can't Sleep," *Consumer Reports*, January 14, 2016, www.consumerreports.org/sleep/why-americans-cant-sleep/.

If a lack of sleep is affecting your health and robbing you of happiness, try these suggestions. And if you still find yourself fighting a losing battle with insomnia, don't hesitate to contact your doctor. Don't be embarrassed; insomnia can be a serious issue that fully warrants medical attention.

Smart Ways to Sleep Better

If you wake in the middle of the night and can't get back to sleep, you might have sleep-maintenance insomnia. Try not to stress about the situation. Keep your bedroom lights low—or use a book light—and read a chapter of a book or a magazine article. Say a prayer or recite a soothing psalm. Then try to go back to sleep. I recommend going "old school" with nighttime reading materials, because for some of us, reading on an electronic device can devolve into surfing the web, texting, or reading email.

Make your bedroom a sleep-only zone.

Don't make your bedroom double as your office. And try to avoid watching TV or streaming shows in your bedroom—at least at night. The more stimuli and stressors you invite into your bedroom, the greater the chances one of these things will keep you awake at night.

Have a (virgin) nightcap.

A caffeine-free drink, such as chamomile tea, can help you drift off to sleep. And as tempting as it might seem, try to avoid alcohol in your bedtime drink. Yes, it might knock you out, but alcohol tends to have a rebound effect that will wake you up a few hours later.

Go dark, go cool.

Keep your bedroom cool and dark. If your room is too hot, your sweaty body will toss and turn all night. And if your room isn't dark enough, your senses can be fooled into triggering your internal alarm with the message, "It's morning! Time to get up!"

Bathe your insomnia.

Not all sleep experts agree on the benefits of a soothing bath before bed, but for some people, the warm water—and maybe some scented bath beads or aromatherapy candles—is the perfect prelude for a night of heavenly slumber.

For even more tips, visit www.sleepfoundation.org and www.sleep association.org.

Slow me down, Lord. Ease the pounding of my heart by the quieting of my mind.

COWBOY PRAYER

49

Know When to Call It a Nap

Were you feeling a little skeptical as you read the previous chapter? I don't blame you. Sometimes we can employ all the tricks and tips for better sleep, but then reality sets in. Many of us have jobs that simply don't allow for hitting the pillow at the same time every night or controlling our sleep environment. This was often my experience in the military, and working as a private contractor for the military brings the same challenges.

Perhaps you travel constantly because of your job or other circumstances. Your world is full of different time zones, different cities, and different beds.

The United States is becoming more and more sleep deprived. That's one reason I am trying to bring napping back. A timely 20-minute nap may not be the complete solution for a sleepless nation, but it will improve our mood, alertness, and performance. And I should note that if you nap, you are in good company. Winston Churchill was a noted napper. So were Albert Einstein, Thomas Edison, Margaret Thatcher, and Napoleon. Napping is nonpartisan. Ronald Reagan and George W. Bush napped regularly, as did John F. Kennedy and Lyndon B. Johnson.

Athletes also understand the value of adequate rest and sleep when it comes to one's mental and physical stamina. Basketball great LeBron James sleeps up to 12 hours a day during the NBA season. Steph Curry, star of the reigning NBA champion Golden State Warriors, cites regular naps as part of his recovery process during the season. Olympic gold medalist Shannon Miller noted that her daily naps were as important to her success as any other facet of her training. And two-time NBA Most Valuable Player Steve Nash took a nap every game day.

As for the science behind napping, you might be aware of the landmark NASA study on napping first published in 2005. The study focused on the benefits of napping for commercial airline pilots. According to Mark Rosekind, one of the study's authors, "Naps can maintain or improve performance, physiological and subjective alertness, and mood. A 26-minute nap improves performance in pilots by 34 percent and alertness by 54 percent."[1]

> "Naps can maintain or improve performance, physiological and subjective alertness, and mood. A 26-minute nap improves performance in pilots by 34 percent and alertness by 54 percent."
>
> —DR. MARK ROSEKIND

Dr. Rosekind occasionally gives speeches on the science of sleep. He tells his audiences that it's fine if they nod off during the talks.

If you're feeling groggy, I hope this chapter has you thinking about how to incorporate a nap into your daily routine. I highly recommend the occasional 20-minute nap to boost your short-term alertness and job performance. For most people, a short nap can provide significant benefits without leaving you feeling groggy or interfering with your nighttime sleep later on.

A bit of background on why napping can be so beneficial to many people. Most mammals are polyphasic sleepers. They sleep for short periods of time throughout the day. (If you have a pet, you know exactly what I'm talking about.) However, we humans are monophasic sleepers. Our days are divided into two periods, one for sleep and one for wakefulness. No one is sure whether this is our natural pattern. After all, young kids and elderly people tend to nap regularly. And in some cultures beyond the United States, napping is part of the daily routine.

[1] Cited in Nick Littlehales, "Time Out," in *Sleep: The Myth of 8 Hours, the Power of Naps, and the New Plan to Recharge your Body and Mind* (New York, NW: Hachette, 2017), ch. 5.

But whatever the case, when we don't get enough sleep in the portion of time designated for that purpose, we suffer on a variety of fronts. For example, most of us know that driving while sleepy is extremely dangerous. The National Highway Traffic Safety Administration estimates that drowsy driving is responsible for more than 70,000 auto accidents annually.[2]

If you drive a lot, please be aware of how you are feeling. If you become drowsy while driving, please find the nearest rest area and take a quick nap. If this simply isn't possible, drink a caffeinated beverage. As you might remember from an earlier chapter, I am not a huge fan of energy drinks, but they aren't likely to do as much harm as an automobile accident!

Not everyone will become nappers, but I urge you to consider it. And maybe sleep on it.

[2] Centers for Disease Control and Prevention, "Drowsy Driving: Asleep at the Wheel," November 7, 2017, https://www.cdc.gov/features/dsdrowsydriving/index.html.

50

Age Is Just a Number

*Surely your goodness and love will follow me
all the days of my life.*
PSALM 23:6

Old age is always 15 years older than I am," goes the famous adage. Whatever "old" is to you, it's a place you're in no hurry to reach. People fear how age will affect them mentally and physically. They can't imagine being as happy as they are now when they're "old."

People fear sharp declines, especially when it comes to health and fitness. They also fear that exercise and changes to their diet might hurt more than they help.

But I am here to tell you that I know a lot of people in their AARP years who are healthy, happy, and still challenging themselves physically, mentally, and spiritually.

Older people are generally just as happy as younger people, if not more so. Many senior citizens report a serene sense of satisfaction with life. Further, what is possible at various ages is continually being redefined. Consider...

- Swimmer Dara Torres was still winning Olympic medals at age 41 (while competing in her fifth Olympic Games).
- Actress Susan Sarandon didn't receive the first of her three Academy Awards until age 45.
- Mike Flynt, a grandfather, played linebacker on a college football team at age 59.
- Walt Stack completed the grueling Iron Man Triathlon at 73.

- As this book was heading to press, 45-year-old Texas Ranger pitcher Bartolo Colón was still doing just fine (with an earned-run average under 5.0) as the oldest player in major league baseball.
- Claude Monet was still painting masterpieces well into his seventies.
- George Foreman won the world heavyweight boxing championship at 45.
- Grandma Moses took up painting in her seventies. By the time she passed away at age 101, she had been a world-class artist for a quarter of a century. She was featured on the cover of *Life* magazine at age 100.

Today, advances in nutrition and medicine keep doors of opportunity open wider and longer than ever before. Couple these advances with the experience and wisdom that come with age, and you have a formula for success, health, and happiness that defies "old" stereotypes.

Examples like the ones above and a variety of studies and surveys point to one ageless fact: Age is simply unrelated to one's level of personal happiness.[1]

Scientists have tried to identify common elements among some of the longest living people in the world, many of whom have lived past 100 with a high quality of life. Here are a few of the characteristics they have reported:

- They exercise regularly and consistently.
- They eat a nutritious diet, avoiding highly processed foods and consuming plenty of fresh fruits and vegetables.
- They drink lots of water.
- They avoid loneliness. Relationships within their communities with neighbors, family, and friends are vital.

---

[1] Kamel Gana et al., "Does Life Satisfaction Change in Old Age: Results from an 8-Year Longitudinal Study, *The Journals of Gerontology* 68, no. 4, July 2013, https://academic.oup.com/psychsocgerontology/article/68/4/540/569189.

- They practice and enjoy regular sex—usually with their spouse, who is their longtime partner in a mutually monogamous relationship.
- They live with and depend on their extended families, who offer cradle-to-grave security and support.
- They emphasize relationships and harmony over the pursuit of wealth or success.
- They avoid loneliness.

Note how many of these characteristics mirror what we have been exploring in this book.

- They avoid highly processed foods. In fact, virtually none of their food is highly processed.
- They eat a nutritious diet. They don't overeat, and their diet is high in fiber, whole grains, nuts, and "good" fats. They tend to avoid salt, saturated fats, and refined sugars.
- They drink lots of water.
- They consume plenty of fresh fruits and vegetables.
- They avoid loneliness. Relationships within their communities with neighbors, family, and friends are vital.
- They practice and enjoy regular sex—usually with their spouse, who is their longtime partner in a mutually monogamous relationship.
- They live with and depend on their extended families, who offer cradle-to-grave security and support.
- They emphasize relationships and harmony over the pursuit of wealth or success.[2]

When you arise in the morning, think of what a precious privilege it is to be alive—to breathe, to think, to enjoy, to love.
MARCUS AURELIUS

[2] Cited in Walter Larimore, *God's Design for the Highly Healthy Person* (Grand Rapids: Zondervan, 2003), 64-65.

51

Don't Let Your Job Make You Sick

Choose a job you love, and you will never
have to work a day in your life.
CONFUCIUS

At work—it's where you'll spend the lion's share of your waking hours (and maybe a few of your sleeping hours as well). You might find yourself spending more hours on the job than you spend with your significant other, your family, or your friends. You might even spend more time working than sleeping.

Consider this: If you begin a full-time, 40-hour-per-week career at age 22 and retire at 65, you will devote the equivalent of 3,440 24-hour days to your job. That's 9.5 round-the-clock years' worth of nothing but work. No vacations, no holidays, no sick time. And no sleep.

This information isn't meant to depress you. It's to help you appreciate a simple fact: Your job is a significant personal investment of your time and energy. So choose your career path wisely. Don't chase the money or prestige at the expense of personal satisfaction and fulfillment or physical and emotional health. Reread the quote by Confucius above and let those words sink in.

> Don't chase the money or prestige at the
> expense of personal satisfaction and fulfillment
> or physical and emotional health.

Given all that we invest in our jobs, it's worth considering how our jobs are contributing to our health and well-being—or lack thereof. If your job provides wellness benefits of any kind, that's great. Make sure you take advantage of them. If not, try making a few suggestions.

Many of us don't feel like we have a lot of job options, but I encourage everyone I know to take a long, clear-eyed look at how their jobs are affecting their health. And I have taken my own advice.

Several months ago, stress was beating me up. I felt like an MMA fighter battling a larger and much more experienced opponent. Not all of the stress was related to my job, but a lot of it was. I wasn't making enough money, and I was dealing with a boss with multiple personalities, most of them toxic. I felt more like a prisoner than an employee.

I was still trying to work out and eat healthfully, but I had no appetite—yet I was putting on fat. I was miserable.

So I decided to take the advice I had given so many others. I knew I had to make some changes in my life. The first thing I did was quit my job. Then I decided to change my attitude about finances, and I started to work on two of the books I'd been promising myself I would write. This book is one of them.

The result: My stress was substantially reduced. It didn't go away completely, but my attitude improved, I started to sleep better, and the fat started melting off.

This is why I encourage you to do all you can to ensure your job contributes to your overall health. I am happy to see so many companies, large and small, providing health- and wellness-related benefits to their employees. And if your job is damaging you in any way, please know that you are not really stuck. You're not stuck unless you want to be.

As we close out this chapter, let's consider a few famous people's career paths.

Gerald R. Ford—model turned US president

Dean Martin—steelworker turned entertainer

Golda Meir—schoolteacher turned prime minister

Howard Cosell—attorney turned broadcaster

Tim Green—NFL lineman turned novelist and attorney

Babe Ruth—bartender turned baseball player

Boris Karloff—Realtor turned horror flick actor

Clark Gable—lumberjack turned actor

Paul Gaugin—stockbroker turned artist

Steve Martin—magician turned comedian turned actor turned bluegrass musician and author

Albert Einstein—patent-office clerk turned physicist

Mike Reid—pro football player turned country music star

Vitali Klitschko—pro boxer turned Ukrainian political leader

Ina Garten—nuclear policy analyst turned cookbook author and Food Network host

Margaret Thatcher—chemist turned prime minister

John Grisham—lawyer turned bestselling author

10 Rules for Ensuring a Case of Job Burnout

1. Drive yourself to make more money, faster, than your coworkers.

2. Eat sporadically. Skip breakfast and replace as many meals as possible with a caffeine- and sugar-loaded energy drink.

3. Try to work up at least one hefty rage a day. Always give full vent to your anger and frustration.

4. Worry about everything. Don't meditate or pray or reason about anything.

5. Don't take vacations. They're for wimps.

6. Ignore minor physical ailments, such as abdominal pain, indigestion, or insomnia. They're probably nothing, and who has time to go the doctor anyway?

7. Always stick to your opinions like superglue. Don't even entertain the notion that you could be (gulp!) wrong.

8. Never delegate responsibility. Do it all yourself so that you get all the credit.

9. Sleep four or five hours a night. Wear those bags under your eyes like little puffy medals of honor.

10. Do not, under any circumstances, relax and enjoy your successes. If you let up, someone might pull ahead of you.

52

Slowww It All Down

Roberts Wesleyan College professor Dr. Joel Hoomans notes that the average person makes about 35,000 "remotely conscious" decisions every day. He adds that about 225 of these are about food.[1]

If you're like me, you might be skeptical about that number. Other estimates put the number of *conscious* decisions at 612 per day. But whatever the case, our brains do a lot of decision work every single day. Our senses take in billions of bytes of information every second, and consciously, subconsciously, and semiconsciously, we are forever processing that input and responding. Or deciding *not* to respond.

This is why our minds need a rest, a respite, just as much as our bodies do—if not more—but it's hard to give ourselves permission to seek that rest. Maybe this will help: If you believe, as I do, that we are created in God's image, you should note that God rested for one-seventh of the process of creating the whole world. That's 14.29 percent, in case you're really into stats. This seems like permission to me—and a good reason to shake the myth that we must be in constant motion to be productive (and, therefore, important).

Many preachers and teachers exhort us, "Bear fruit!" However, one of the fruits that our lives are meant to produce is peace. Look around you at work. Do you see many peaceful people? Do the same thing next time you are on a plane or in the middle of your morning commute. Do you see peace abounding, or do you see frantic, frustrated people all around you?

---

[1] Joel Hoomans, "35,000 Decisions: The Great Choices of Strategic Leaders," *Leading Edge Journal*, March 20, 2015, https://go.roberts.edu/leadingedge/the-great-choices-of-strategic-leaders.

Set yourself apart from the harried hordes by reminding yourself that resting your body and your mind is an important part of the process of living. Give yourself permission to slow down. From time to time, take your time. Look at something beautiful. Listen to something beautiful. That is not wasted time—that is spending time wisely.

The word "rest" appears 508 times in the NIV translation of the Scriptures. The word "peace" appears 249 times. That's way more than many of us might think. It's almost as if the One who created our minds and bodies knows a few things about how we can function best. Constant stress and constant activity for its own sake are destructive. We need times of rest, recovery, and renewal. Restoration is good stewardship. It's not lazy or wasteful; it's wise.

Sometimes we view life as a race when it should really be a journey, one that's leading in the right direction. Take some time to consider whether your journey is bringing you closer to what (and who) makes you feel most alive.

Let's remember that speed isn't everything. It takes a glacier a year to move as far as you can walk in five minutes. But eventually, glaciers carve canyons and move mountains. Slow movement can change the world. Patience and perseverance can change the world. So can you.

Rest in these truths for a while.

Is it possible that peace exists inside of us but our minds are too loud to hear it?

Matt Dragon

53

Believe You Can Do It!

have a love/hate relationship with the cliché "Believe in yourself." As I have said many times in this book, I am a huge fan of positive self-talk, of a winning attitude. However, like many clichés, "Believe in yourself" can be taken too far. Way too far sometimes. Believing yourself to be a capable person is a good thing; believing you are incapable of ever making a mistake is elevating yourself so high that you're due for a painful fall.

> Believing yourself to be a capable person is a good thing; believing you are incapable of ever making a mistake is elevating yourself so high that you're due for a painful fall.

The key is finding a balance between deifying yourself and dismissing the voices telling you that you're not talented enough, smart enough, or strong enough to succeed in life. That you will never get in shape. That you will never eat more healthfully. That you will never stick to a new lifestyle.

I encourage you with all my heart to develop a sense of resolve. You are worth the effort. The people in your life are worth the effort. They want you around. They need you around. And they want you to be at your best. Firm resolve keeps our chins up and our eyes looking forward even in the face of inevitable setbacks.

Speaking of setbacks, did you know...

- Retailer R.H. Macy endured seven failures before his famous New York store finally caught on.

- Author Theodor Geisel saw his first children's book rejected by 27 publishers. Today, we know Geisel by another name—Dr. Seuss.

- Baseball legend Babe Ruth struck out 1,330 times en route to his 714 home runs.

- English novelist John Creasey received 753 rejection notices before he published the first of his 564 books.

Imagine the moments of doubt each of these individuals endured. But they never gave in to that doubt.

Whatever goals you have set in life—health related and beyond—a solid, reasonable belief in your ability, a faith in your calling in life, and a passion for what you are doing will make your efforts successful. And you'll enjoy your efforts much more as well.

In several interviews, businessman and former NBA star Magic Johnson said his attitude and mindset toward battling HIV have been just as important to his health and sense of well-being as the medications he has been taking for decades now.

Regardless of your age, ethnicity, or profession, a strong belief in yourself and a sense of optimism will increase your life satisfaction by almost 30 percent—making you happier and more successful in your personal and professional lives.[1]

One of the techniques that helps me strike a healthy balance between self-confidence and self-aggrandizement is what I call grateful exercising. This exercise is simple. I lie in bed or on the couch and simply meditate on everything I am grateful for. I try to do this after I work out. I give thanks for the ability to take action to improve myself. I give thanks simply for being alive.

I also do grateful exercising every night before I go to sleep. It helps put my day, my whole life, in perspective. It helps reset my priorities. It recharges me spiritually and emotionally. It helps me rest more peacefully with a hopeful heart for tomorrow.

---

[1] J. Lounsbury, J. Loveland, E. Sunderstrom, and L. Gibson, "An Investigation of Personality Traits in Relation to Career satisfaction," *Journal of Career Assessment* 11, no. 3 (2003): 287-307.

I have found that being grateful for my blessings helps me avoid becoming prideful about them. It helps me be confident without being cocky. As Oswald Chambers wrote in his classic devotional *My Utmost for His Highest*, "We cannot do what only God can do. And He will not do what we can."

This mindset is key to being confident yet grateful stewards of the minds and bodies God has given us.

54

Screen Your Screen Time

Imagine going to a restaurant and ordering almost everything on the menu. When the food arrives, you nibble at a few of the dishes, decide you don't want any of some others, and completely devour one or two. Then you waddle away from the restaurant overstuffed, frustrated, and poorer in both money and time.

No sensible person would feed his stomach this way, especially if he is trying to lose some weight and be a healthier person. However, this is how many of us feed our minds with TV and other forms of electronic media. We watch, not necessarily because we are hungry for entertainment, fulfillment, or information, but simply because it's there. Watching TV becomes a hobby. (How often do you park yourself in front of the TV or the laptop because it's something to do rather than to watch something in particular?)

This approach can lead to incessant channel surfing (or channel-guide surfing) in a quest to find something that holds our interest. It's possible to spend more time trying to find something to watch than to watch an entire program or movie.

Psychologists have discerned that some people watch so much TV that they lose some of their ability to engage in a conversation. Watching TV is passive, they note, and can lure people into a "sit back and be entertained" mode. Many of us believe the same thing can happen with excessive use of one's smartphone, tablet, or laptop.

Next time you walk into a room with a TV, challenge yourself to avoid turning it on except to watch a show you really want to see or something you have recorded digitally. Then use the newfound hours you'll have to do something meaningful with family or friends, get some work done, exercise, or read your Bible or a favorite novel. Actively participate in life. Don't let passive screen gazing gobble up too much of your time.

> Actively participate in life. Don't let passive screen gazing gobble up too much of your time.

You might be aware of the 2017 TED Talk by psychologist and marketing professor Adam Alter. During this talk, which has received more than three million views, Alter noted how we are spending more and more of our free time staring at screens. Further, he reported an alarming dichotomy. We feel good about apps that focus on relaxation, exercise, reading, and health. Apps like this tend to increase our happiness level. On the flip side, we feel less happy when we use apps centered on dating, social networking, gaming, entertainment, and general web browsing. But here's the punch line: "We're spending three times longer on the apps that don't make us happy," Alter reported. "That doesn't seem very wise."[1]

It's fascinating how Alter's findings mirror what P. Wu found in his doctoral research at the University of Michigan in the late 1990s. Wu found that watching TV excessively can *triple* one's desire for more material possessions while at the same time reducing personal contentment by 5 percent per every hour of TV watched daily. Do the math, and you'll have a proven formula for increased happiness.[2]

So let's all try to be smarter about our screen time. If we do, we'll experience one of life's best gifts—hours of time that we can invest in the things that truly matter.

---

[1] Adam Alter, "Why Our Screens Make Us Less Happy," TED Talks, April 2017, https://www.ted.com/talks/adam_alter_why_our_screens_make_us_less_happy.

[2] Cited in David Niven, *The 100 Simple Secrets of Happy People* (San Francisco, CA: HarperSanFrancisco, 2001), 14.

55

Accept Yourself First and Then Better Yourself

*Accept one another, then, just
as Christ accepted you.*
ROMANS 15:7

If someone asked you, "Who are you?" how would you respond? Some people define themselves by their job title, their bank account balance, or the carefully maintained image they see in the mirror before going out in public.

But none of these things capture a person's true essence. And all of them can lead to a fundamental dissatisfaction with life—the continual striving for a more prestigious job title, a fatter bank account, or a more appealing reflection in the mirror.

Every New Year, millions of people make resolutions related to self-improvement. Many of these focus on getting in shape (or getting *back* in shape).

Of course, I wouldn't be writing this book if I didn't want to encourage people to be their healthiest selves. However, there is a delicate balance here. We need to be grateful for all that God has given us. We need to accept ourselves as worthwhile human beings. We acknowledge that yes, we have faults, but we are basically good people. Generous people. Good spouses, siblings, and friends.

I hope that all of us can look in the mirror and see someone who, every day, does way more good than harm. That realization is a strong foundation for unleashing your efforts to be a healthier person. I'll explain what I mean.

If you are down on yourself, giving yourself all kinds of negative messages, that might provide temporary motivation to start eating better, exercising, or getting more sleep. But over the long haul, that kind of self-talk—"I'm fat and ugly" or "I'm helplessly addicted to junk food"—won't inspire you to strive for better health. That's negative motivation. It's living in fear and self-loathing.

I urge you to think more positively. Your self-talk should include statements like these:

- "I'm a marvelous creation of God, and my lifestyle should reflect this fact."
- "God has good things planned for my life, and I want to be healthy enough to experience them fully."
- "I need to take better care of myself when it comes to rest, relaxation, and rejuvenation. I'm worth it, and so are the people God has placed in my life."

I want to emphasize that accepting yourself doesn't mean becoming complacent or refusing to grow as a person. Instead, it means you appreciate your own value, and that value becomes the catalyst for self-improvement. It's all about positive reinforcement, not negative reinforcement.

Those who have studied self-esteem have found that people who accept themselves can take defeat and disappointment in stride rather than letting these things destroy them. They refuse to be defined by life's inevitable failures. This applies to failures on the job as well as in the gym or at the dinner table. Let's strive to see setbacks merely as obstacles to be climbed over.

Unhappy people make a practice of magnifying each defeat to monstrous proportions. They identify with each failure. They believe the failure is a sign of more to come. Instead of saying, "I fell short of my goal," they tell themselves, "I am a failure. I'll always be a failure."[1]

Think of the close friends or family members in your life. These people aren't perfect. They've made mistakes, they've faltered in their paths from time to time, and they've probably even hurt you somewhere along the road. But you still accept them and value them. Shouldn't you do the same for yourself?

> One of the greatest moments in anybody's developing experience is when he no longer tries to hide from himself but determines to get acquainted with himself as he really is.
>
> NORMAN VINCENT PEALE

---

[1] J.D. Brown and K.A. Dutton, "The Thrill of Victory, the Complexity of Defeat," *Journal of Personality and Social Psychology* 68 (1995): A 712-22.

56

Laugh a Little—or a Lot!

Our mouths were filled with laughter,
our tongues with songs of joy.
PSALM 126:2

In this book, I have shared dozens of ideas about strengthening existing health habits and adopting new ones.

As we near the end of this journey, I want to urge us to develop and maintain a sense of humor. What does this have to do with our health and well-being? How about this: Adults who have a sense of humor outlive those who don't find the humor in life. In a now-famous study, the medical school at the Norwegian University of Science and Technology studied 54,000 adult subjects for seven years. At the outset of the study, the subjects noted their ability to find humor in everyday life and expressed their views on the importance of a sense of humor as a coping skill.

As the study progressed, researchers found that the greater the role humor played in one's life, the greater the chance of his or her survival. The people who scored in the top 25 percent for humor appreciation were more than 35 percent more likely to be alive at the end of the study than those in the bottom 25 percent. (The study took into account such variables as the subjects' general health, age, gender, and lifestyle.)

In a subgroup of 2,015 subjects who had a cancer diagnosis at the beginning of the study, results indicated that patients who had a strong sense of humor had a 70 percent higher survival rate than those with a poor sense of humor.

Sven Svebak, who headed the study, noted that previous research has indicated that humor helps people deal with stress and maintain a healthy immune system during stressful times. "Humor works like a shock absorber in a car," he said. "You appreciate a good shock absorber when you go over bumps, and cancer is a big bump in life."[1]

The Norwegian study has been supported by other research over the years. It is common knowledge that a healthy vascular system is key to a long, healthy life, and a University of Maryland study showed that while stress decreases blood flow in the body, experiencing humor increases blood flow by 22 percent. Imagine what a good laugh could do for your workout?

I know people who work out on their treadmill or elliptical while watching *The Office* or some other humorous show on TV. I know others who listen to a favorite humor podcast while running or walking.

William Breitbart, psychiatry chief at New York's Memorial Sloan-Kettering Cancer Center, offered yet another insight on why laughter is good medicine for the body and soul. He notes that someone who can see humor in the side effects of treatment like chemotherapy might be willing to endure the treatment longer, "and that could be a way that humor affects survival."[2]

Here is even more evidence that humor and getting healthier go hand in hand. Did you know that 100 laughs a day provides a cardiovascular workout equal to about 10 minutes of rowing or biking? And there's more happy news: Laughter stimulates stress release in the same way exercise does. Laughter also helps fight infection by sending into the bloodstream some hormones that reduce the power of stress to weaken the immune system.

Further, in a study of hundreds of adults, the ability to laugh—at oneself and circumstances—was found to be an important source of

[1] Sven Svebak et al., "A 7-Year Prospective Study of Sense of Humor and Mortality in an Adult County Population," *International Journal of Psychiatry in Medicine* 40 (2010): 125.

[2] Cited in Sebastien Gendry, "Life Expectancy: A Laugh a Day May Keep Death Further Away," American School of Laughter Yoga, March 13, 2007, http://www.laughteryogaamerica.com/learn/research/life-expectancy-laugh-day-death-662.php.

life satisfaction. In fact, people who enjoy silly humor are 33 percent more likely to feel happy than those who don't.[3]

It looks like research is revealing what Solomon knew thousands of years ago: "A cheerful heart is good medicine" (Proverbs 17:22).

I travel throughout the United States and around the world, and I see people who face a variety of pressures from school, work, family, finances, and the like. What's more, we are flooded with more information (from a wider variety of sources) than we can handle.

In other words, sometimes you might feel like a nuclear reactor that is melting down. Laughter is the safety valve that can prevent disaster. So don't become so caught up in life's demands and stressors that you can't lighten up and loosen up once in a while. Laugh at life's absurdities rather than letting them get under your skin. Seek out the comic relief provided by humorous books, TV shows, YouTube clips, and other media. Look for the humor in various situations, and strive to be a source of laughter and good humor wherever you go. There's no denying it—life is hard and stressful. But if you can maintain your sense of humor, you can have the last laugh.

I'm not surprised that some of my favorite athletes and coaches have great senses of humor. It helps keep life in perspective, especially during times of challenge, large and small. For example, I enjoy following NFL quarterback Carson Wentz on Twitter. A while ago, he found himself locked in a gas station bathroom (never a good thing). But here's what he tweeted about it: "Just got locked in a bathroom at a NJ gas station. Praise the Lord for the attendants w/ the garden shears, & the other guy w/ the leg kick."

Here's another example: Pat Williams is senior vice president for the NBA's Orlando Magic. If you follow basketball, you know that this team has struggled in recent years. When asked to comment on his team's woes, Williams responded, "We can't win at home. We can't win on the road. I just can't figure out where else to play."

[3] Erik Barker, "The scientific proof that laughing is really good for you," *The Week*, September 8, 2016, http://theweek.com/articles/646149/scientific-proof-that-laughing-really-good.

It's not surprising that in addition to being a basketball executive, Williams is a sought-after motivational speaker. I get the sense that his sense of humor helps his team endure even during hard times. And there is research to back this up.

> It seems logical that creating a fun environment would be likely to enhance enjoyment levels, but in addition to this, it appears that coach-athlete interactions and integrating activities that athletes perceive as enjoyable may also have a positive impact on preparation and, ultimately, performance. Preparing fully, in any context, is difficult to do if we are not enjoying the journey we are on. When we are experiencing an element of pleasure, we tend to push ourselves harder, focus more, and have a greater overall sense of satisfaction.[4]

Indeed, King Solomon was right. Laughter is good medicine, and it's available without a prescription. So fill up.

Laughter is an instant vacation.

MILTON BERLE

---

[4] Warrick Wood, "Is It Important for Athletes to Have Fun?," *Psychology Today*, May 12, 2016, https://www.psychologytoday.com/us/blog/the-coach-athlete-relationship/201605/is-it-important-athletes-have-fun.

57

Set Your Mind to "Productive"

This book has been quite a journey. Thank you for sticking with it. Living a healthier, more mindful life isn't easy. New information pours out every day. Some of it is solid research and some of it is just hype, but in any case, we can feel like we are in a constant state of information overload as we try to keep up with it all. It's possible to feel burned out.

Here are a few tips on developing a mindset that will help you live a healthier life and gain more control of your health.

Be Offensive

By this, of course, I don't mean that you should go around trying to offend people. Instead, I am talking about knowing your priorities and operating accordingly. You should wake up every morning with a purpose and a plan. Don't let your email inbox or your voice mailbox rule your day. Don't spend all your time putting out other people's fires. Focus on where you need to be and how you will get there. Some people are successful in their efforts to get healthier while others are not. The difference starts in the mind.

Be Selfish About Your "Me Time"

Even if you are an extreme extrovert, you need some time alone. It's vital to the rest/recover/recharge process. You need time to think, pray, and meditate. (This is one reason I devoted a whole chapter to solitude.) Many of us wake up every morning to hundreds of emails, a swarm of family demands and responsibilities, and the latest crisis on social media. Yes, some of these things need our attention, but we all need time to ourselves. I've noticed that my healthiest friends and family members find time, virtually every day, to be alone. And when they cannot find the time, they *make* the time.

> Even if you are an extreme extrovert, you need some time
> alone. You need time to think, pray, and meditate.

It's okay, for example, to say things like, "Let's reschedule our business dinner for a half hour later. I'll be more productive and more engaged if I can get a little time to decompress."

Disconnect from All the Tech

Remember chapter 45, where we considered taking a techno-fast? Technology can stress us out and wear us down. Imagine you're a musician who is never given time to warm up before a performance or never given an intermission or any kind of break between songs. Or imagine you're a basketball player, but your team isn't allowed to warm up, call time-outs, or regroup and strategize at halftime. Whatever your endeavor, if you have to be "on" all the time, you will burn out.

Continue Mastering Your Craft

I have a friend who is an amazing golfer even though he's in his late fifties now. He can't drive the ball as far as he used to, but he's shooting scores just as low as when he was 30. The reason is, he approaches golf like a kung fu master. He understands that his muscles and reflexes aren't the same as they once were, so he is forever learning to adapt his game to the changing dynamics. Because of this, his scrambling and his sand saves are better than they have ever been. Likewise, we might need to modify our exercise regimens, our diets, or even our relaxation techniques as we get older or experience other life changes, but we can always strive to be our healthiest selves.

Conclusion

Thank you for reading this book. I truly appreciate your taking the time to explore ways to get healthier and stay healthier.

I believe the ideas I have shared can work for you. They have worked for me and for many people I have coached, trained, worked out with, and advised over the years. If you sat next to me on an airplane, you would probably hear me talking about what's in this book because it's what I am passionate about. I am still excited about working out and training. I am passionate about learning what's new in the worlds of nutrition and stress reduction. I have learned to love learning. I hope you share this mindset.

From time to time, people tell me, "Your advice is too simple." But this isn't really a criticism to me. I *want* my ideas to be easy to understand and implement. Besides, simple does not mean easy.

In this book, I have shared what I have learned and practiced for the past 26 years. It certainly wasn't easy to be consistent for more than a quarter of a century, but it was simple. I plan to keep learning and to keep striving for better health for the next 26 years—and beyond. Will you join me in this quest?

I'm ready to take my own advice and go for a long walk now, so let me close with this. I hope that as you read this book, you took some action. Maybe you added a healthful food or two to your shopping list. Maybe you decided you would try a techno-fast. Maybe you stopped reading midchapter to take a walk.

I encourage you to keep the momentum. Keep doing things to make your life better. And please share your success stories. Write a review or leave a comment at harvesthousepublishers.com. Whenever I learn that I have helped someone get even a little bit healthier, I feel like the nerdy kid who gets asked for a date by the most beautiful girl in the school.

I pray that God will do things in your life that make you feel that way too.

Live passionately. Live hopefully.

To learn more about Harvest House books and
to read sample chapters, visit our website:

www.harvesthousepublishers.com

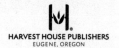

HARVEST HOUSE PUBLISHERS
EUGENE, OREGON